ULTIMATE LAP-BAND SUCCESS

The Support Surgeon's Guide to Getting the **Most** From Your Gastric Band!

DR. DUC C. VUONG

ULTIMATE LAP-BAND SUCCESS

By Dr. Duc C. Vuong

ISBN: 978-0-9822206-3-4
Library of Congress Control Number: 2009926452

Published by Escalation Press
Cover and Interior Design by Nathan Brown,
Writers of the Round Table Inc.

ACKNOWLEDGEMENTS

First, I would like to personally thank my patients. I learn so much about myself from each and everyone of you. As you make strides in your lives, I see how much more I could do with mine.

I would also like to thank my office staff and their cruel task master, Sheri Morris, my nurse program coordinator. They do all of the dirty work that makes me look good, and our accomplishments as a clinic would not be possible without their dedication.

I want to thank my father, whose courage provides me with constant inspiration, even to this day, even after his passing.

Lastly, I want to thank my life partner, Melissa, who willingly edits my poor grammar and, sometimes to my dismay, openly questions my authority. She has also provided me with my greatest accomplishment to date—our baby girl, Kizzie.

CONTENTS

The Perioperative Phase 1

Preoperative Lap-Band Knowledge Test 4, 16

Lap Band Nutrition 6, 25

How Do You Know When To Stop Eating?. 8, 29

Social Eating With The Lap-Band 10, 38

What is My Happy Weight?. 12, 45

Refocus Your Focus 14, 51

The Maintenance Period 58

Weight Loss Slow Down, a.k.a. Weight Loss Plateau. 60, 64

Healthy Shopping Skills 62, 74

Holiday Eating Tips 83

Top 10 Realistic Resolutions That Will Make a Difference 89

Final Thoughts. 95

Resources 97

Photos 100

About the Author 104

Section One

The Perioperative Phase

During the past few years, as I have been developing a comprehensive bariatrics program, I have become known as the "Support Surgeon." (Personally, I think the title is kind of catchy.) I have acquired this name for several reasons, but primarily because I consider support groups to be more important than the actual gastric banding surgery itself. In my clinic support groups are not optional, and my patients attend several, even before surgery. Following surgery, my patients abide by the rule that I will not adjust their band unless they have attended a support group that month. I personally lead group three times per week in my clinic, so patients have plenty of opportunities to talk with fellow patients, meet with me and my staff of weight loss specialists, maintain motivation, and learn better strategies.

I am currently conducting a study comparing my clinic against another clinic, and the early data show that my patients average a significantly better weight loss. I can't ascribe this to any superiority in operating skill, since the surgery itself is straightforward and the other doctors are quite excellent surgeons. Our working hypothesis is that my patients' consistently high levels of success are directly related to their regular participation in a comprehensive support program. More importantly, we are trying to ascertain if my patients will be significantly "happier" patients in the long term, but as you can imagine, quantifying "happiness" is no easy task.

I've traveled around the country to lead support groups for other surgeons and their patients, and I help clinics and hospitals set up their own complete support programs based on my own best practices. Unfortunately few places offer a comprehensive support system, and my goal is to change that soon. So I guess "The Support Surgeon" title is befitting.

In this section, I have included the worksheets and discussion topics that I cover in my key support groups. I require all of my band patients to attend six perioperative sessions, one per week, two groups before and 4 groups after their surgeries. This means that patients will come to my office for at least six weeks in a row initially! I personally lead these sessions, because I believe these topics are critical for a Lap-Band® patient's success and happiness. They then must attend monthly maintenance support groups, where we discuss broader issues like "Body Image." This is the minimum requirement, but they are welcome to come every week if they would like.

Even though I am most likely not your surgeon, you can maximize your learning from this book by actively participating in it, as if you were in an actual group at my clinic. Follow these steps to get the most out of this book:

- Answer the questions first. Really write out your answers. Once you have completed the questions for a section, go ahead and flip to the discussion of that topic.
- Take notes as you read along. I hope to offer you many easy-to-follow tips and strategies for maximizing your success. Make lists of what you will incorporate into your lifestyle now.
- Go back and review your answers after reading the discussion section. This will help emphasize what choices need work or rethinking.
- Teach these tips to someone else. Better yet, have a friend participate with you. You can compare your answers and what you've learned. In essence, start your own support group, using this book as a basis.
- Revisit the questionnaires every couple of months. You can see what changes you have adopted and set new goals. Then reread the discussion section to see if there are more things you can change to help keep you on track to a healthier body.

My patients often revisit support groups that focus on their trouble spots, like "Social Eating With the Band." They will come back a month or a year after their first participation in that session to reinforce their knowledge of good band eating habits. So hang on to this book once you've completed it.

I also offer live DVD recordings of my actual support groups that I have led. If you are interested, please visit *www.MoreFromMyBand.com* or email me at *morefrommyband@gmail.com*. You can also visit me on Facebook at Dr. V's Gastric Band Group.

Now let's get started!

Preoperative Lap-Band Knowledge Test

1. With the Lap-Band, I will be able to eat
   a. Anything I want right away.
   b. All breads and meats.
   c. About 1100 - 1200 calories a day.

2. Immediately after surgery, I will
   a. Wake up skinny.
   b. Have some discomfort that should get better gradually.
   c. Go on a long trip.

3. With the Lap-Band, I can
   a. Drink all the alcohol I want and expect to lose weight.
   b. Eat all the ice cream I want and expect to lose weight.
   c. Have sweets (if I do it in moderation) and expect to lose weight.
   d. None of the above.

4. I should
   a. Keep my weight loss efforts a secret.
   b. Tell everybody I am having Lap-Band surgery.
   c. Understand that social support is very important to my long-term success.

5. When eating with a well-adjusted Lap-Band,
   a. I should eat only liquids so it goes down easy.
   b. I should try to eat small amounts of nutritious foods.
   c. I should take one last bite after I feel full just to be sure.

6. I need to start an exercise program
   a. Before surgery.
   b. After surgery.
   c. Never! Exercise is a bad word.

7. After I get my Lap-Band
   a. I don't need to do anything further. The hard part is done.
   b. Go on a cruise to celebrate my "journey" that everyone talks about.
   c. Continue to attend support groups and get regular check-ups and adjustments.

8. Name three (or more) sources of protein.

   _____

   _____

   _____

   _____

Lap Band Nutrition

1. What is the First Rule of Lap-Band Eating?

2. Give an example of where this rule applies.

3. How many calories per gram of Protein? Carbohydrate? Fat?

4. How many calories per gram of EtOH (alcohol)?

5. Why is this relationship important?

6. What is the problem with mixed drinks?

7. Give one rule about salad.

8. What are Empty Calories?

   _____

   _____

   _____

9. Give 3 examples of Empty Calories.

   _____

   _____

   _____

10. Write one poor eating habit that you have ALREADY changed since your weight loss surgery:

    _____

    _____

    _____

    _____

11. Write one poor eating habit you NEED to change:

    _____

    _____

    _____

    _____

How Do You Know When To Stop Eating?

1. How many times a day SHOULD you eat after the Lap-Band surgery?
    _____
    _____

2. How many times a day DO you eat now with the Lap-Band?
    _____
    _____

3. If the answer to #2 is different from #1, write down WHY you think they are different.
    _____
    _____
    _____
    _____

4. Now that you have the Lap-Band, how do YOU know when you are full?
    _____
    _____
    _____
    _____

5. What happens to you if you ignore that signal?
    _____
    _____
    _____
    _____

6. If something gets "stuck" what should you do?
    _____
    _____
    _____
    _____

7. What should you NOT do if food gets stuck?

_____

_____

_____

_____

8. One more time: What is the First Rule of Lap-Band Eating?

_____

_____

_____

Social Eating With The Lap-Band

1. What is the First Rule of Lap-Band Eating?

    _____

    _____

    _____

2. Write down one situation where this rule applies in a social setting.
    (Really write it down, rather than just think about it. That's what these
    worksheets are for!)

    _____

    _____

    _____

    _____

    _____

    _____

3. After your Lap-Band, how will ordering food be different?

    _____

    _____

    _____

    _____

4. What about drinking before and with dinner?

    _____

    _____

    _____

    _____

5. What is the problem (or problems) with alcoholic drinks?

    _____

    _____

    _____

6. What is one strategy for keeping on track if you decide to splurge at an upcoming party?

    _____

    _____

    _____

    _____

7. Do you want to learn to cook, or re-learn to cook?

    _____

    _____

    _____

8. Remember, if you do what you've always done, you will get what you've always gotten. So when it comes to socializing, what is one thing you will commit to changing?

    _____

    _____

    _____

    _____

What is My Happy Weight?

1. What do I mean by Ideal BMI? What do I mean by "Happy Weight?"
    How are they different?

    _____

    _____

    _____

2. If you have already decided, then what is your Happy Weight?

    _____

    _____

    _____

3. How did you arrive at your number for your Happy Weight?

    _____

    _____

    _____

4. Write down three things you can do to achieve your Happy Weight.

    _____

    _____

    _____

5. Do you know of anyone who undermines your efforts to reach your
    Happy Weight? If so, what can you do to get this person to be more
    supportive?

    _____

    _____

    _____

6. What is an activity you will do with friends/family other than social eating?

    _____

    _____

    _____

7. What is one thing you will change right now to make yourself happier?

_____

_____

_____

8. POP QUIZ: What is the First Rule of Lap-Band Eating?

_____

_____

_____

Refocus Your Focus

1. Regarding food, what did you do prior to weight loss surgery?

    _____

    _____

    _____

    _____

2. Regarding family, what were your relationships like prior to your weight loss surgery?

    _____

    _____

    _____

    _____

3. Regarding work, what was it like prior to your weight loss surgery?

    _____

    _____

    _____

    _____

4. How did you spend your weekends prior to weight loss surgery?

    _____

    _____

    _____

    _____

    _____

5. How did you spend your family time? Name one activity you did together.

    _____

    _____

    _____

    _____

6. Name one charity for which you would like to volunteer and why.

    _____

    _____

    _____

7. Write the first sentence of your journal entry for today.

    _____

    _____

    _____

8. Do you keep a food diary?

    _____

9. Name one thing that is different in your life since your surgery.

    _____

    _____

    _____

10. What is one thing about your life that you will change right now?

    _____

    _____

    _____

Preoperative Lap-Band Knowledge Test

1. *With the Lap-Band, I will be able to eat*
   a. *Anything I want right away.* There is perioperative swelling around your gastroesophageal junction (GEJ) where your surgeon had to do the dissection to place your band. It is not possible to predict the amount of swelling that your body will experience nor exactly how much pressure the band will put on your stomach. So I always keep my patients on a high-protein liquid meal-replacement program, like Optifast® or Smart Forme®, for one week after surgery. This is to prevent any food from getting stuck. If food gets stuck, you will vomit. If you vomit, your band is more likely to slip.

   b. *All breads and meats.* This is different for every patient. Some patients can eat bread and some can't. Some can eat steak but not chicken. Some used to be able to eat eggs but after an adjustment can't any longer, at least not until the next adjustment. There are no rules about how an individual's body will react; it is absolutely unpredictable. I think it probably has more to do with psychological and mechanical eating factors than it does with the band itself.

   c. *About 1100 - 1200 calories a day.* Once a band is well adjusted, this should be your caloric intake that will keep you feeling full IF you eat real food and do not take in empty calories. You could have a well-adjusted band and consume 1100 Calories with just one McDonald's milkshake. What is "real food?" Think…Caveman! This is a tip that I learned from Dr. Kevin Prentice from Dallas. He is a chiropractor but knows a lot when it comes to healthy eating. He says to think like a caveman when you are making food choices, and eat only what a caveman would quickly recognize as food. A caveman ate fresh meat, fruit, vegetables, and grains. For each choice you make, ask yourself, "Would a caveman recognize this as food?" He would recognize a potato, for example, but not a potato chip, so put the potato and not the chips in your shopping cart. Real food is not processed and does not come in shiny packages. It is usually located on the outer edges of supermarkets. Another way to tell if something is real food is if it comes with either no list of ingredients (e.g. an apple) or if you recognize all the ingredients listed on its packaging.

2. *Immediately after surgery, I will*

    a. *Wake up skinny.* We all wish this, but we know it just doesn't work that way. Most of you have struggled for years with your weight, so you can't expect it to go away overnight!

    b. *Have some discomfort that should get better gradually.* The perception of pain is different for every patient, but many studies have shown that pain experience is significantly less after laparoscopic surgery compared to traditional open surgery. Return to work is also faster. Patients can also have a referred pain to their shoulders. If pain persists longer than normal, beware, as this could be a sign of something wrong.

    c. *Go on a long trip.* Immediately after surgery, travel is not recommended. Not only could you develop blood clots in your legs from sitting still too long, but most patients don't really know enough about "life with the band" to make the trip enjoyable. They may be scared to eat at all, and become hungry and anxious, or they may fill up on margaritas, and become malnourished and ill.

3. *With the Lap-Band, I can*

    a. *Drink all the alcohol I want and expect to lose weight.* This is my patients' favorite subject! I know they are tired of hearing me go over this every week, but here we go…1) How many calories per gram of protein? Answer=4. 2) How many calories per gram of carbohydrate? Answer=also 4. 3) Now, how many calories per gram of fat? Answer=9! In other words a chunk of fat has more than twice the calories of a chunk of carbs or protein. If you can't remember the numbers, that's ok. It is the ratio that is important. Another way to look at it is that for the same amount of calories, you could eat more than twice the amount of carbs or protein. Here is the punchline: 4) How many calories per gram of alcohol? Answer=7! Everybody knows how bad fat is at 9 calories per gram, but many don't realize that alcohol is right below it at 7. There have been many banded patients who have lost weight and put it all back on with alcohol. Much of the time, alcohol is consumed along with highly caloric mixers, making a margarita top 600 calories. If you have a problem controlling your alcohol intake, please seek professional help. Get a handle on this before having weight loss surgery; otherwise, no weight loss surgery will work for you.

b. *Eat all the ice cream I want and expect to lose weight.* Despite what Einstein might have thought about simple interest, I think ice cream is the most powerful force in the universe. The band has no chance against it. I have enjoyed a bowl of ice cream on special occasions, but if a whole tub of ice cream has comforted you in the past, do not fool yourself into thinking that "just a taste" will be ok. That taste will turn into a lot more. And remember, the band works by controlling appetite so that you consume fewer calories; it does not erase the high calories in ice cream or other treats.

c. *Have sweets and alcohol (if I do it in moderation) and expect to lose weight.* This is the most debated question in my clinic! Here is my stance. If I am ever called to testify about this in court, I will say to the judge, "Judge, I swear I told them never to eat sweets and never to drink alcohol." But the truth is there will always be special occasions, vacations, and celebrations. You just have to be aware of the temptations and acknowledge the choices that you are making. If salty chips are your downfall, then don't believe that you can stop with just one and don't buy a big bag of them to tempt you. The types of decisions you will need to make in order to be successful with the band will become clear by understanding yourself through deep self-exploration and honesty.

d. *None of the above.*   This is the correct answer. I think the difference between C and D is OFTEN the reason people hit "Weight-loss Plateaus," a concept that we don't believe in at my clinic. In other words, if I had to guess, MOST people who can't "get off the last 20 pounds" or "have stopped losing weight for no apparent reason" would probably answer C to this question, and perhaps they need to redefine what "moderation" means or (even better) cut out all sweets to see the last pounds drop. But I'm sure a few would answer D, and something else is the culprit. There is always an answer to why you've hit a plateau, whether it is physical, emotional, or psychological.

4. *I should*

a. *Keep my weight loss efforts a secret.* Have you ever dieted in secret? How did that work out for you? Let me guess — not so great! That's probably because the people around you expected you to stick to your established patterns and offered you your favorite foods or urged you to indulge at your favorite restaurants. You had no one to talk with when the diet became difficult to maintain, nobody knew anyway, and so you probably quit. We encourage our patients to find their support people and enlist their help.

b. *Tell everybody I am having Lap-Band surgery.* I wish every one of my patients would shout, "I had my Lap-Band surgery by Dr. Vuong!" but the truth is having weight loss surgery is a private decision. If you are not ready to share your surgical experience with people you know, then you can try to say things like, "I'm just trying to make better choices!" Hopefully they will be respectful of your new lifestyle and encourage you to be healthier.

c. *Understand that social support is very important to my long-term success.* Our society is built around food and eating. Everybody has an Aunt Patty who says, "I knew you were coming so I baked you your favorite - pecan pie!" Aunt Patty is not trying to sabotage your weight loss efforts but rather is trying to welcome you into her home. If you don't let Aunt Patty know about your new lifestyle beforehand, in this situation you will either unhappily undermine your weight loss or upset your relative. In order to have long-term, meaningful weight loss happiness, you must have social support, which is why I recommend that my patients tell everyone about their surgery.

5. *When eating a with a well-adjusted Lap-Band,*

    a. *I should eat only liquids so it goes down easy.* The band is not designed to stop liquids. In fact if liquids can't go down, then you are in a lot of trouble! Eating only liquids is not a long-term option, and consuming too many calories in the form of liquids is an easy trap to fall into. I consider ice cream, refried beans, and other soft and fatty foods to be liquids because they are not stopped by the band and add far too many calories to your diet. Many people do not meet their weight loss goals because they are unwilling to give up high calorie drinks (including alcohol). You've got to decide which you want more—to be healthier and thinner or to have that soda. Diet sodas are not an option either. Study after study has shown that people who consume the most diet sodas also tend to be the heaviest. This is in part because the chemicals in the diet soda accustom our palate to unnaturally sweet flavors, meaning that they encourage us to consume more sugar overall. And soda, diet or not, provides you with absolutely no nutrients. Read the ingredients – do you recognize many of them as food? Some people think that shakes are good, and while it is true that high protein, low-calorie shakes have their role in the life of a banded patient, shakes should not be relied upon for lasting weight-loss happiness. We want you to learn to eat and enjoy real food again.

    b. *I should try to eat small amounts of nutritious foods.* The happy banded patient should eat 3 small, nutritious meals a day, and diabetics should add a healthy snack. But what is "nutritious"? This is where learning to read labels comes in handy. A simpler way of thinking about this is to give your food the caveman test (see #1). For example, chicken is nutritious and a caveman would recognize a roasted bird. He would definitely not recognize chicken nuggets or the containers of sauce to dip them in. So choose the chicken that's been grilled or roasted, but leave behind the battered, processed, sauced-up varieties.

c. *I should take one last bite after I feel full just to be sure.* "One last bite" gets a lot of bandsters into trouble. Learn to listen to the cues that your band gives you to stop eating, and yes, these cues will change over time. They are dependent on when your last adjustment was, what size band you have, how high your surgeon placed your band, etc. If you feel satisfied, you are done and there's no need to eat more.

6. *I need to start an exercise program*
    a. *Before surgery.* It is likely that you need to think of "exercise" in a whole new way. Understand that for most bandsters, starting an exercise program before surgery just means increasing your activity level. You can do this by parking further away, walking around the office, using the stairs instead of the elevator, taking out the trash once a day instead of telling your kids to do it, etc. Do not waste your time purchasing expensive exercise equipment or gym memberships! And if you haven't run in 15 years, you will be miserable if you try it immediately.

    b. *After surgery.* Waiting until after surgery is not ideal, but it is better than nothing. You can always start by just implementing the small daily tips listed above and others you may think of. As you lose weight, you will probably feel up to longer stretches of activity at greater intensity.

    c. *Never! Exercise is a bad word.* Remember how joyous it was to run, jump, roll, climb, dance, and delight in all sorts of movement as a kid? You didn't think of it as exercise then, and you certainly didn't think it was awful. Try to think like a kid again and find activities that raise your heart rate that you enjoy. You'll probably be able to do more and enjoy moving more as you become healthier. This is an exciting time to rediscover old interests that got you moving around, or discover new hobbies, like playing frisbee with your kids or grandkids or gardening. Once you rethink the concept of exercise, you can develop a more systematic approach.

"Physical fitness" is different from "daily activity" and has been shown to extend lifespan and improve overall quality of life. Physical fitness is accomplished by a regular exercise regimen that is designed to stimulate your heart rate to a goal target rate about 3 times a week. It also includes resistance work with weights. A local gym or college often provides affordable personal trainers who can help design a safe and convenient program for you to improve your physical fitness. But by increasing your level of daily activity, you will also be improving your level of physical fitness, so don't wait. Get started now!

7. *After I get my Lap-Band*
    a. *I don't need to do anything further. The hard part is done.* The surgery itself is only about 10-20% of the process. The other 80-90% of it is YOUR dedication and commitment to making those small daily changes that are necessary for long-term success. I have heard of many patients who are unhappy with their band because they either never lost their desired weight or lost it and regained it all because they never changed the choices they made. If this is your situation, try to find a convenient support group for banded patients to help get you back on track. You can also find lots of resources or useful links on my website *www.MoreFromMyBand.com*.

    b. *Go on a cruise to celebrate my "journey" that everyone talks about.* If you can find the right program, then the Journey will be a fantastic one! But a wise man once said, "The journey of a lifetime starts with one step." So be prepared to make that first post-surgery step. This means having your social support in place, finding the right program, increasing your daily activity level, making better choices, and just being happier. Consider postponing that cruise until you've become more familiar with your new life with the band.

c. *Continue to attend support groups and get regular check-ups and adjustments.* This is EVERYTHING when it comes to long-term weight loss happiness. Communicate with your physicians, surgeon, nurses, and fellow bandsters. Learn new strategies, commiserate about your challenges, delight in your successes, and keep on top of your health. It's a whole new day, baby!

8. *Name three (or more) sources of protein.*
    Meats, Fish, Poultry, Soy products, like tofu
    Beans, Cheese, Dairy, Nuts

Notes

Lap Band Nutrition

1. *What is the First Rule of Lap-Band Eating?*
    Protein First. This means that at each meal you should eat protein before you eat carbohydrates or fat. If your answer was "Chew, chew, chew" or "Don't drink during meals" or "Eat until mush" or something like that, I will say that those are indeed some good guidelines that you need to know. But make no doubt about it: the First Rule is Protein First. Most patients' problems with weight loss and the band can usually be traced back to the violation of this rule.

2. *Give an example of where this rule applies.*
    This means that you have to wait until your "main dish" or "meat dish" arrives! What happens when you go to a Mexican restaurant, for example? They bring out chips and salsa, of course! "Protein First" means that you have to pass on the chips and salsa. "Protein First" means you have to say no to the warm, hot bread that many restaurants bring you after you order. "Protein First" means you have to pass on salads. It means that when you are waiting to be seated at a restaurant, you cannot try the bar nuts. You have to wait until your protein comes before you eat.

3. *How many calories per gram of protein?* 4
    Carbohydrate? 4
    Fat? 9

4. *How many calories per gram of EtOH (alcohol)?*
    7

5. *Why is this relationship important?*
    See Lesson #1, Preoperative Lap-Band Knowledge Test, Question #3 for more details, but basically it means that you can eat more than twice the amount of protein or carbohydrates as you can of fat for the same amount of calories. It also means that those alcoholic drinks can add a lot of calories (and no nutrients) to your intake without helping you feel full.

6.   *What is the problem with mixed drinks?*

Two words: simple syrup. Do you know how to make simple syrup? Equal parts sugar and water. In other words: boil 1 cup of water, then add 1 cup of sugar and dissolve. That's it. This is the main ingredient in mixed drinks, often labeled as "syrup" or "mixer," which means that they are full of sugar and its calories. Another question: how many calories in a margarita? The average sized margarita can pack around 600 calories, depending on the mixer they use! We know that liquids go right through the band. And we know that you can't ever have just one margarita. You buy yourself one, then your friend buys you one, and before you know it, you've had 3 or 4. This means 2400 calories, or more than twice the amount of daily calories for a well adjusted Lap-Bandster, in drinks alone! There have been many determined and well-intentioned bandsters, who either lost weight and then put it back on or "plateaued" and can't lose anymore, all because of mixed drinks. It's ok to have mixed drinks on occasion, but you've got to understand the choice you're making. I tell my patients, "Avoid all fruity drinks, especially the ones that come with those little umbrellas."

7.   *Give one rule about salad.*

Everyone thinks that salad is a healthy choice, but as a bandster, it is very important that you unlearn this. SALAD IS NOT A BAND-FRIENDLY CHOICE. In the first place, it violates the number one rule of Lap-Band eating: Protein First, since salad is served first. But here are a few other reasons to avoid it on a regular basis and tips for doing so.

- Most salad is VERY LOW in nutrition. The plain iceberg lettuce that is the foundation of many salads is mostly water and some fiber, which can be tough on a band.
- If you choose a salad, the greener and darker the better. Choose the mixed field greens or spinach salad.
- Eat the tomatoes. They are high in a nutrient called lycopene that may help lower certain cancer risks.
- The salad dressing can pack a big caloric punch! Choose the vinaigrette if possible. Avoid the creamy and cheesy ones, like ranch, buttermilk, or peppercorn, that are very high in fat. Even their low-fat versions still have a lot of calories.

- If you just can't give up ranch dressing, then ask for the dressing on the side and use just a little bit.
- Ask them to bring the salad with the main meal and eat your protein first. Chances are, you won't feel like eating the salad afterwards.
- Ask if you can substitute the iceberg salad for something else with protein in it, like bean salad.

8. *What are Empty Calories?*
    They are the scourge of every Bandster. Empty calories are foods that are rich in calories but poor in nutrition. They are the usual culprits when I hear or read about a "weight loss plateau."

9. *Give 3 examples of Empty Calories.*
    Ice cream, soft drinks, candy bars, chips, and nearly every highly processed food that resides in a snack machine. I would even say most fast foods! Their low nutritional value does not justify their high caloric counts. Sadly, they are often the most convenient foods. A small "snack" from the machines at work can take just seconds and a few coins to purchase, but may contain a few hundred calories that come mostly from sugar.

(No answers are provided for #10 and #11.)

Notes

How Do You Know When To Stop Eating?

1. *How many times a day SHOULD you eat after the Lap-Band surgery?*
    I recommend that my patients eat at least 3 small meals a day, with each meal containing some protein (remember the First Rule?). I also tell my diabetics that they should add a fourth small snack in the afternoon to keep their blood sugars level, and by "snack" I do not mean candy, cookies, or other such sweet snacks. A small yogurt or banana would do great!

2. *How many times a day DO you eat now with the Lap-Band?*
    I have a patient who is a dedicated employee and often gets to work early. Like most, she never ate anything for breakfast. She then would work through lunch and by the time she got home in the late evenings, she would be ravenous! Of course, then she would overeat on calorie-dense foods like pasta or fast food. After she got the Lap-Band, she told us that the band was not keeping her satisfied, she was hungry all day, etc. After we went through her daily food intake, we discovered that she still patterned her meals the same way, but now because of the band, she could no longer eat a large amount in the evenings -- thus her constant hunger! We reiterated the importance of eating small meals. I instructed her to have a convenient protein shake and small banana on her drive to work, a small meal for lunch like tuna fish, then dinner when she got home. She voiced understanding of the importance of proper eating throughout the day, but continued to make excuses for her inability to "find time" due to her "hectic work schedule." To this day, I don't think she has made those changes and therefore has not been as successful as she had hoped.

I often tell my patients that I am probably the only person in their lives, much less a doctor, who will tell them to eat more not less. It comes down to quality of food and timing.

3. *If the answer to #2 is different from #1, write down WHY you think they are different.*

Many patients, who expect the band to perform miracles, never change or are unwilling to change their eating behaviors. Needless to say, these patients often are disappointed with their weight loss or find themselves stuck on a "weight loss plateau," a concept that we do not believe in at my clinic. While it is true that if you do not consume enough calories, your body's metabolism will slow down and thus hinder your weight loss, I think this rationale has been grossly exaggerated. The truth is that the vast majority of patients who are not losing weight are consuming too many empty calories. And it is very hard to resist calorie-dense foods if you go too long between meals and become famished.

For example, I have a patient who eats anything chocolate when she is stressed, and I mean anything. Well, in September 2008, Hurricane Ike blew right over my practice and house. It also damaged many of her rental properties. Needless to say, this really stressed her out, and she put on a lot of weight. But to her credit, she came back to our support groups and talked about her weight regain and stress. After a couple of weeks she revealed how she used chocolate to alleviate her stress (she ate anything chocolate every night), but she could not see the connection between this empty calorie consumption and her weight regain. I gave her the tip that instead of consuming lots of whatever chocolate she could find, she should become a chocolate connoisseur and eat only the most expensive and finest chocolates. I told her there were entire online communities and books about fine chocolate. She took my advice, and the following week had limited her chocolate consumption to only one evening and one portion of a very expensive chocolate bar. She lost 2 lbs that week! I was delighted that she was able to find a way to incorporate this passion/ addiction/stress-management-technique into a much healthier approach. I was even happier when she gave all of the credit of this success to talking about it in support group.

Most things I hear or read about from patients (whether it is "I'm too busy," "I can't find time to cook or exercise," "I can't get time off from work," etc.) boil down to one thing: it's all EXCUSES. As mean as that sounds, it's the truth. You are not the busiest person in the world (rather, you choose not to be as efficient in your work as you could be). You are not the most stressed out person in the world (are you more stressed out then, say, our thin and fit President?). You are not the world's worst cook (there are marinated chicken breasts at the grocery that you just pop in the oven) or cannot exercise because of arthritis pain (there are many forms of exercise that do not require stress on joints). These are just excuses that are used to justify not having to make a change. There are tips and techniques to accommodate ALL of these reasons. YOU just have to decide that YOU want to be healthier and happier more than you want that cookie or an hour of television.

Let's go through some useful tips meal by meal. Remember that your goal is to fill your band pouch with the most nutritious food you can.

BREAKFAST: Some patients complain of difficulty swallowing in the mornings. This is thought to be due to the thick mucus that builds up during the night. Try to alleviate this by drinking a cup of hot tea to break up the mucus. Nonetheless, some patients insist that they just "can't eat breakfast." I always ask them exactly what they mean by breakfast. The response usually is, "I can't eat pancakes with syrup and bacon and potatoes, etc." And I say, of course not! The concept of a "meal" is different after band surgery. You will not be able to eat a Denny's Grand Slam Breakfast anymore. But then why would you want to? That is a meal high in calories and fat and low in nutrition. It is too bad that meals like it have come to represent the American breakfast when there are many better options.

I recommend that my patients have a small, sensible breakfast, and always pass on the syrup. If they can't do that, then I recommend that they drink a high protein shake (like Optifast® or Smart Forme®), understanding that this will pass right through their band into the stomach, and then (and this is the key) they must fill their pouch with something nutritious like a yogurt, unsweetened applesauce, 1/3 of a banana, or nutrition bar. The protein shake will ensure that they get their protein, and the real food will help them control their hunger.

LUNCH: Your employer is usually required by law to give you a lunch break—30 minutes in most states. This is your right! Take it, and use it for lunch rather than errands, because it will mean everything to your success. You MUST eat lunch. I can't stress this enough. I really believe that it is by far the most important meal of the day, despite how I just insisted you eat breakfast. If you have a job where you don't get a lunch break, make sure to keep some healthy and easy-to-eat foods handy, like a banana or a sandwich, and eat them a few hours after your breakfast. Surely you can find a few minutes to take a few bites.

Prepare your lunch the night before if you can and bring it with you to work, so that you will be sure to have a nutritious meal handy. If you say that you don't have time to make your lunch, then I ask you, "Aren't you worth the extra 10 minutes it would take?" If you choose to go with coworkers out to lunch, suggest a healthier restaurant choice. If they won't change their plans, don't go. Or, if you do go, then make a healthier choice by focusing on a low-fat, high-protein selection. Look for the "light and fit" portion of the menu.

DINNER: Learn to cook real food! This means buying fresh ingredients, including fresh vegetables, fruits, and meats. Anything you make is better than anything you are going to purchase from a fast food restaurant. There is one caveat to this: it has to be fresh. If all you have to do is pry open a can or tear open a cardboard box and heat it in the microwave, you are probably not making the best choice. Refried beans from a can are usually no better than refried beans in a Tex-Mex restaurant. If it has shelf life, I don't consider it REAL cooking. (Think back to the caveman.) I don't care if it says Lean Cuisine or Healthy Choice on the box—that's all advertising, and don't fall for it!   Learn 5 simple recipes with fresh ingredients and start from there. Watch cooking shows, read magazines, or pick up a cookbook from a bookstore.

If you already know how to cook and currently prepare all of your meals, take time to re-evaluate the techniques you are using in the kitchen. It is not ok to think that you are being healthy if you serve steamed broccoli but then cover it with a thick cheese sauce or if butter is your main ingredient for flavor. But honestly, for most of my patients who are cooks, it's all about portion size and second helpings. Practice eating on a side plate and using a child spoon or fork—at least initially until taking small bites becomes second nature.

4. *Now that you have the Lap-Band, how do YOU know when you are full?*
Most patients report experiencing a "pressure feeling" right in the middle of their chest. They are confused by the location of this feeling. I tell them that that is where their band is sitting. Many are often surprised to learn this. So I explain it like this: Most surgeons will use a liver retractor to access the gastroesophageal junction (GEJ) so that they can place the band. If you look at your surgical scars, you should have a small scar in the upper middle, where both sides of your rib cage come together at your sternum or "breastbone." If you put your finger on this scar move up one inch, then imagine a line going from your finger to your back, you will hit your band. Yes, your band is that high up! And that is why you get the pressure feeling in your chest and not around your belt line like before.

Some patients report feeling pain in their shoulder blade or back. This is for the same reason. I have one patient who gets a small burp that is her signal to stop eating. I have several patients who will hiccup—this is probably due to irritation of the diaphragm muscles when their pouch is full.

While these signals are convenient, not everyone gets them. But don't be disappointed if you don't have a signal or haven't recognized it yet. It is so much more important to learn the feeling of SATIETY. It is OK to be satisfied. (It's what Mick Jagger has been looking for all these years.) Stop eating when you are satisfied, not stuffed. This is often the most difficult part for many patients, many of whom do not know what it means to be satisfied. If you eat regular meals, you have no reason to become stuffed, because you'll eat again in a few hours. Overeating is often a way of compensating for going far too long between meals.

5. *What happens to you if you ignore that signal?*
    It's like what Clubber Lang, a.k.a. Mr. T, told the reporter in Rocky III: "Pain." And there is not much that you can do about it. If you overeat once with the band, I bet you will not do it again, as long as you stay well adjusted. If you never go back for an adjustment, the fluid in the band will very slowly seep out over the years, and it will be as if you've never even had the surgery.

6. *If something gets "stuck" what should you do?*
    Most patients say waiting works. It will usually pass within 2-5 minutes. Walking around helps. Getting up helps. Some websites mention Productive Burps or "PB's." This is where you belch the food particle back up, and it is usually accompanied by a slimy film. I think it is just a nice way of saying "vomiting without retching."

I teach my patients to never let themselves get into this situation in the first place. You can do this by taking small bites, chewing thoroughly, taking your time, and stopping when you are satisfied.

After the food piece has cleared, you must not eat another bite of this meal. Don't save it and try eating it for dinner--you're just not ready for it. You have to back down to the next lower food texture. For example, if chicken gave you trouble, then you have to back down to fish, which is easier to chew. If red meat was the culprit, stick to chicken for a while. Give your body 2 or 3 days before you try again. If it gets stuck a second time, avoid it all together. Resign yourself to the fact that you might not be able to eat that food for a long time. But don't worry, it won't be forever.

Also, don't mix up your food. I had one patient, a very nice and well-intentioned fellow, tell me once that rice got stuck. I had him explain what he ate to me. He said he had made an Asian-style meal with thinly sliced beef, broccoli, and rice; but when he ate the rice, it gave him trouble. Probing a little further, he explained to me that he had placed all of the ingredients into a big bowl and mixed them together. And I said, "So you picked out one item at a time? You ate the broccoli, waited, and then ate the beef?" He sort of lowered his head, realizing his mistake, and said, "No, I put a little of everything on my fork and ate it."

This is problematic for a couple of reasons. First, he doesn't know which food item was the culprit. Was it really the rice, like he thought? Or was it actually the broccoli or the meat? Because he mixed it all together, there really is no way to be sure. Secondly, if he was able to take a little of everything on his fork, he clearly took too big of a bite! This was probably a lapse back to his old habits. Granted, old habits are hard to shake, but changing them is very important to avoid this sort of problem.

The other cause of food getting stuck that I see is due to over-consumption of alcohol. Patients will have one too many drinks, get tipsy, forget their techniques, and take too big of a bite or not listen to their cues. They get stuck and have a food accident. This can be easily avoided if you will do one simple thing: do not drink any alcohol until after you've eaten all that you are going to eat. Even better, don't drink alcohol.

7. *What should you NOT do if food gets stuck?*
    If food is stuck, chances are it is stuck in your esophagus, which is a long tube connecting your mouth to your stomach. Think of it like your kitchen sink drain.

If something gets stuck, DO NOT DRINK WATER, hoping to force it down. Like your clogged sink, it will only back up and make your life even more miserable. Instead, stand up, walk around, and wait for it to pass. Then don't eat that food item again for at least several days.

8. *What is the First Rule of Lap-Band Eating?*

I know this has been a question earlier in this book, but I can't emphasize it enough. Protein First.

Notes

Social Eating With The Lap-Band

1. *What is the First Rule of Lap-Band Eating?*
    Everybody all at once now: "Protein First!"

2. *Write down one situation where this rule applies in a social setting.*
    This is a very important question. Many people can recite rules by memory easily and some claim to know everything that they are SUPPOSED to do, but many can't actually implement those rules. I don't think it is because they are incapable of understanding the rules, but rather, that they've never been shown how to actually implement these life-changing tips. If you are to be a happy Lap-Band patient, you must understand how to make your band work for you during social situations. I will provide several situations where this rule applies. This list is in no way meant to be complete. Hopefully once you've mastered it, you can add your own examples and share them with other banded colleagues.

    I already mentioned how this rule applies at a restaurant and some strategies for sticking to it. Simply wait to eat anything until your main course arrives. Either do without a salad or ask for it to be served with your entrée and don't have anything from the bread basket. Pass on the chips and salsa. This is a good rule even for people who have not had the band but are struggling with their weight, because it is easy to consume several hundred calories before the main course arrives.

    At a party this rule would mean that you should avoid the snacks and appetizers that circulate. Since this is very hard to do when you are hungry, try to eat before going to a party or an event that features a buffet. And what should you eat before going? Protein! Have a chicken breast sandwich or piece of fish. Then you can probably resist the appetizers or sample one small snack at the party and not be tempted to fill up on what are often high-calorie treats. Another trick is to keep a glass (of sparkling water, for example) in your hand. That will keep you from feeling awkward while everyone else has a plate and also make it a difficult balancing act should you be tempted to sample something. And remember that with the band, you should not eat near to the time you drink (see Question #4 below).

Do not make the mistake of "saving" your calories for a party. Not only will you end up eating far more calories (and most likely empty calories) than you should, you will also be at risk of having food get stuck. That's definitely not something you want to have happen in a crowded room!

Of course, if no one knows why you suddenly are not eating their food, they may try to pressure you into eating more than you want or should. You can either tell them about your surgery or politely insist that you are trying to make healthier choices and that your restraint is in no way an insult!

3.   *After your Lap-Band, how will ordering food be different?*
     When I ask banded patients this question, most say that they now order off the appetizer portion of the menu, immediately take half of their food home, or do not order anything at all but rather just share some of their spouse's or friend's meal. While these are all great, there are two more things that I want my patients (and you) to understand about life after Lap-Band surgery.

     It is ok to throw food away. You do not have to clean off your plate. Forgive yourself for breaking this well-ingrained American familial law. After you are banded, it should be impossible for you to consume all of the food on a typical plate in one sitting. I say SHOULD because there are ways around everything, and what is "filling" will change depending on where you are in your adjustment cycle. Many of us were raised hearing that we could not go play until we'd cleaned our plate. Now feel how liberating it is to leave some food behind and go do something else!

     You have to try different types of food. I often say, "If you do what you've always done, you will get what you've always gotten." Since you are trying to change your health, it is best to change your habits, which can be a fun experience! There is such a bountiful assortment and variety of food for us to experience in this country. But sadly, I can count on one hand what most of the people who seek my help eat on a day-to-day basis. They usually go to the same 3 or 4 restaurants and usually order the same 3 or 4 items. For me, this is just not that interesting of a way to eat. We love food in our clinic, and we want our patients to learn to love food again, too! You might want to visit different grocery stores or shop at a local farmer's market to load up on fresh produce. Pull yourself out of your eating and shopping rut and experience new flavors at least a couple of times a week.

4. *What about drinking before and with dinner?*
    Most patients know the "Do Not Drink 30 Minutes Before or 30 Minutes After You Eat" rule, but most do not think about how this applies in social situations. First let me explain the origin of this well-known rule. It was started by Dr. Paul O'Brien, one of the great Lap-Band forefathers from Australia. He told me that he used to tell his patients not to drink one hour before and one hour after eating! At the same time, he told his patients that it was good to drink a glass of red wine, because as we all know, wine is meant to be consumed with meals in order to compliment the flavors of the food. Patients complained, however, that they were confused by these two guidelines: one said not to drink for 2 hours, and the other said to drink wine in order to augment the meal. So Dr. O'Brien compromised and created the 30-minute rule. As you can see, it is rather arbitrary, but it is grounded in good intentions.

    The thinking behind this rule is that liquid will push food through your band faster and thus negate the purpose of the Lap-Band, which is to have real food sit in your pouch and create a sense of satiety. But I am not sure that this "rule" has ever been validated. I will leave it up to your own personal experience to determine its efficacy (some patients swear by it), but if you prefer not to risk overeating, then just stick to the rule.

5. *What is the problem (or problems) with alcoholic drinks?*
    As I've said earlier, a regular margarita can pack up to 600 calories. These

are not good calories either, but rather empty calories (they provide you with no nutrients). Calories aside, other pitfalls abound.

Many times in social situations where alcoholic beverages are served, less than ideal snacks are also being served. Take your average Super Bowl Sunday, for example. Think about all of the tempting deep-fried finger foods, hamburgers, chips, dips, candies, sweets, etc. All of these things can wreak havoc on anyone who is trying to make healthier choices. Alcohol lowers our inhibition, and we are far more likely to throw caution to the wind after a couple of beers. Most of us can recall a personal experience in which alcohol made us act a little more freely than usual. And when people around us are overindulging, it becomes even harder to resist. I am not suggesting that you will never have another alcoholic beverage again or never be able to attend another Super Bowl party. I am just stressing the importance of understanding the choices that you make, and if you accept and prepare for the consequences that come with that choice, then you will be well on your way to successful long-term weight loss.

6.   *What is one strategy to keeping on track if you decide to splurge at an upcoming party?*
Socializing is just a part of everyday life. It is neither healthy nor realistic to think that the key to dieting success is to "avoid all parties." Celebrations happen, and you should be able to take part in the festivities of graduations, anniversaries, holidays, weddings, reunions, bat mitzvahs, sweet sixteen's, you name it. You just have to understand the choices you make regarding those occasions.

Here is the key: if you are going to CHOOSE to SPLURGE for that occasion, it is imperative that you make up for those extra calories, not the day before or 2 days before or even 3 days before, but the ENTIRE WEEK before! This is the guideline we give to our patients. I insist on this not because I am a cruel despot, but because of the realistic rate of calorie expenditure versus the density of empty calories available at parties (more on this later). And be realistic about whether or not you will splurge; indulging should be a conscious decision and not a spur-of-the-moment impulse. Thinking through the potential pitfalls along your weight loss journey and planning for them will help you to stay on track, but it requires self-reflection and honesty.

7. *Do you want to learn to cook, or re-learn to cook?*
   Why do I ask you (dare challenge you) with this question that seems so simple at first glance? To put it simply, anything you prepare fresh from fresh ingredients is better than anything you buy at a restaurant or get from a can or a box or a frozen meal—yes, even if that box or meal is labeled "Lean Cuisine", "Sugar Free!" "Fat-Free" or "New and Improved." Take a moment and think about what has to go into these processed "food" items in order to give them a shelf-life of weeks, months, and even years in some cases. Some shelf items will outlive me! Is that REAL FOOD? Is that what you really need to be putting into this one-and-only body of yours? Why is it that we will put premium gas or high quality oil in our cars, but we give our bodies the cheapest and lowest quality fuel we can find?

   Most restaurants don't prepare their food on site. Their menu items are usually shipped to the restaurant in huge bags of processed and frozen products that are then assembled in the kitchen. This to me is not real food and definitely not real cooking. And you end up paying a lot more for it in the long run, in terms of your health.

   Cooking is a great way to create lasting, meaningful memories with your family. Get your children involved in the process. This will not only teach them new skills but also ingrain in them an appreciation for the nourishment we put in our bodies. Can't think of how you can do this? Here are a few tips. Have your children help you with the prep work that is age appropriate, like snapping green beans or rolling limes (but also have them help you clean up). Take them shopping at outdoor farmers markets to see all of the fresh ingredients and where they come from. Reconnect with Mother Earth by starting and growing an herb garden or a few vegetables. This is an invaluable opportunity to teach your kids about science and nature and ecological cycles, etc. Before you say, "I don't know anything about science, I hate bugs, or I can't____, can't____, can't____," ask yourself this question: What would I be willing to do if it meant that my children would avoid the same path of weight struggles that I've taken? And it could be fun to learn something new and have an excuse to get out a bit more.

8. *Remember, if you do what you've always done, you will get what you've always gotten. So when it comes to socializing, what is one thing you will commit to changing?*

Don't wait; do it now! Write it down and commit to starting something new! Start with a small change. A simple tip to finding a change that you can stick with: don't give something up but rather ADD something new. Add some walking, add some vegetables, add some quality family cooking time. The more you add, the less time and space you'll have for old, bad habits.

Notes

What is My Happy Weight?

1. *What do I mean by Ideal BMI? What do I mean by "Happy Weight?" How are they different?*

   It is not meaningful to say "I am overweight because I weigh 250 pounds," because there is a difference between a woman who is 5 feet tall and 250 pounds and a man who is 6 feet 2 inches tall and 250 pounds who also happens to be a linebacker. BMI, or Body Mass Index, is a medical term to approximate a person's ideal body weight that factors in height. An ideal BMI is considered to be between 19 and 25; anything higher is considered to indicate being overweight. It is not a perfect measure, but a good starting point. Most of you know your BMI already, but in case you don't, there are many BMI calculators on the internet that are free to use. You can find one on my website at *www.TexasCitySurgical.com*.

   Your Happy Weight, on the other hand, is the weight at which you are not struggling with your relationship with food. You look good, you feel good, and you have a fun social life. You're confident, you're active, and you're out there participating in life. This might be a BMI of less than 25, but it could also be a BMI of higher than 25. It just depends on YOU and YOUR particular journey, and where YOU are at this point in YOUR life. That means that your Happy Weight could change, depending on what you want from your life and your health, but more importantly, what you want to DO with your life. So think about your Happy Weight often.

2. *If you have already decided, then what is your Happy Weight?*

   It's ok if you haven't decided on a Happy Weight, especially early on in your weight loss journey. The important point is that you start thinking about your new life and what it will be like. Some of my patients don't pick a number. Instead they set other measurable goals—like clothing size, medication change, or walking endurance. For example, my early postop patients might say, "I want to fit into a single digit dress size," or "I want to get off my blood pressure medications," or "I want to be able to walk to do my grocery shopping." These are great goals to set!

3. *How did you arrive at your number for your Happy Weight?*

This is a very important question. If you left this question blank, go back and answer it now. You have to understand the motivations behind the decisions you make. What drove you to give the answer you gave? How you derived your Happy Weight is just as important as the actual Happy Weight itself. If you write down that it's what you read some Hollywood actor weighs, then you might need to think more about what you, yourself would be happy with. A motivation that stems from your personal desires will help carry you through the difficult times.

4. *Write down three things you can do to achieve your Happy Weight.*

This should be easy. There are so many resources available to help you with this one. Try books, the internet, e-newsletters, etc. Let me give you a couple of wonderful websites to visit. *www.WLSchannel.com* is the first internet channel completely devoted to the care of weight loss surgery patients. *www.LapBandTalk.com* is an online social site where you can meet and blog with other band patients. For e-newsletters, you can try my website *www.MoreFromMyBand.com.* I write my own newsletters and you can also purchase my books and support group DVD's. A friend of mine, Cher Ewing, a life coach who is also banded, offers a weekly e-newsletter for free at *www.BandedTogether.net.*

In case you need some immediate ideas on how to achieve your Happy Weight, here are a few.

- **Enlist support from your closest friends and family**. Support is everything in weight loss because social interactions are so important to everyday happiness. The people you spend your time with can help you achieve your goals, or they can lure you back into old habits. Getting them on board with your new lifestyle is essential.

- **Add extra, simple activity at work**. Instead of calling your coworker, walk down the hall to deliver the message; instead of rolling in the chair, get up and walk. Stand while talking on the phone. Offer to pick up forms from another building. Without adding much time or effort, you can increase your calorie expenditure by at least 100 calories a day. Many studies have shown that people who constantly "fidget" (tapping their foot or shifting in their chairs) also tend to weigh less. Small bits of movement can really add up.

- **Cut down on alcohol consumption.** Quitting all at once if you are used to regular drinks can be difficult – instead cut back a little more each week. Understand the calorie choices you make when it comes to alcohol.

- **Learn to cook real food or change how you cook.** Remember, anything you cook from real ingredients is better than anything you buy already prepared, even if it says "Weight Watchers" on the box.

- **Start an easy and convenient exercise routine.** Convenience is the key because it reduces the number of excuses you can come up with to avoid it.

- **Change your driving routine to avoid old temptations like donut shops and fast food restaurants.** I had a patient who used to stop at McDonald's every day on the way home from work to get an order of fries. If this sounds like you, then don't drive near the McDonald's. If it's an ingrained habit and you're feeling tired or stressed, it will be hard to resist your old routine.

- **Be happy.** I'm not being a smart-aleck here. If you are enjoying your life and the people you are spending it with, you will achieve your goals more easily.   In fact, this is the main message we try to deliver to our patients—just be happy.

5. *Do you know of anyone who undermines your efforts to reach your Happy Weight? If so, what can you do to get this person to be more supportive?*
It is important to understand who your support people are and how to

communicate this support to them, so take this question very seriously. This is a scary proposition because it means that you might have to acknowledge the fact that someone who is very near and dear to you might be subconsciously (or even consciously) undermining your weight loss efforts. Count yourself lucky if you can only think of one person. Many of my patients have multiple offenders.

You've got to take an honest accounting of those closest to you. Remember the old saying, "Actions speak louder than words." So despite what this person might say, it is more important to determine whether or not their actions are consistent with their words. If someone says they are happy to see you trying to become healthier but then brings home your favorite dessert and eats it in front of you, they are not making your efforts any easier!

It is also important to determine if there is anything that you are doing to contribute to this person's behavior. Are you empowering them to behave this way? If you want them to be more supportive, you have to tell them what you want from them, what type of support you need, what questions to ask or not to ask, what kind words or critical words are helpful, etc. Deep down, they love you and want you to succeed, but you have to let them know how to support you because they can not read your mind and you should not assume that they can or should be able to do so.

And if you determine that they don't really love you or don't really want to see you succeed, then you've got to decide how important it is to keep this person in your life. That is why this question is so scary.

6. *What is an activity you will do with friends/family other than social eating?*
    Social gatherings are a central part of life, but why do we make them all center on food? This world has so much else for us to experience. If you live in the city, your non-food options are almost limitless. Try visiting museums, zoos, planetariums, historical sites, old homes, monuments, etc. Go see plays or go to book readings. Call your local Chamber of Commerce if you are stuck. Join groups with similar interests. There are

walking groups, fitness groups, hiking groups, museum groups, all sorts of groups. There are community classes in watercolor, literature, country dancing, movie appreciation, gardening, almost anything you could possibly want to learn. If you don't live in the city, then don't be discouraged. There are many of the same opportunities in small towns—you just have to look for them. And you probably have more open space for playing Frisbee or birdwatching.

A recent study suggested that the root cause of obesity in America may be that we've lost our connection to nature. I think there might be some truth to this. Plan outdoor games, kick the ball around, take a walk around the neighborhood after dinner, organize a family softball/football tournament, or try fishing or hiking trips. Plant a family garden and make it a criterion to use something from the garden if anyone wants to have a family get-together where food is involved. These are just some tips, but feel free to find your own and share them with me on my Facebook page.

7. *What is one thing you will change right now to make yourself happier?*
Ask yourself, what will make me really happy? It can be as complex as "find a new job that I really love" or something as simple as "be able to walk without my knees hurting." This is a Call To Action! Don't just think about it. Do it! Haven't you waited long enough? Aren't you tired of sitting on the sidelines, watching as life passes by you? Say these three simple words: Enough is enough.

8. *What is the First Rule of Lap-Band Eating?*
Please tell me you know this one by now.

Notes

Refocus Your Focus

1. *Regarding food, what did you do prior to weight loss surgery?*
   Be honest. That is the key to this question. Sometimes our memories fail us. Sometimes we can't face the truth of our bad behaviors and choices we've made in the past. Let me tell you, you're not alone. So that you might find some courage, here are some things my patients have told me. One patient admitted to eating an entire ½ gallon of ice cream in one sitting during stressful times, and she did this regularly. I have patients who admit to eating out 7 days a week. One patient went through the drive thru at midnight on the way home from night shift. One patient could easily drink 10 Diet Cokes a day (remember that diet soda consumption is linked to obesity, even if the sodas themselves have zero calories). Another patient could eat an entire vat of gumbo. One patient hid candy bars around the house, so her family couldn't find them.

   Also consider some of the good choices you may have been making, like trying to eat fresh fruit every day, testing out low-fat recipes, or not allowing chips in the house. If you're reading this book, you are aware that you've made bad choices, but I'm sure you've also made some smart decisions. Just as important as recognizing what we need to change is reinforcing what we've been doing that is healthy.

2. *Regarding family, what were your relationships like prior to your weight loss surgery?*
   What role has family played in your current weight struggles? How far back can you trace it? Were you the chubby child? Were you the thin sibling? What were your parents' attitudes about food, family dinners, and your physical appearance? How did this affect your body image? Did everything revolve around food?

   What is your fondest memory involving your family? Does it involve food? You might be surprised--most of the time it doesn't, and even if food is in the picture it plays a distant second role to the people. When you reflect on these good memories, hopefully you will realize that it is the FAMILY that is important and not the FOOD.

3. *Regarding work, what was it like prior to your weight loss surgery?*

    Face it. We spend anywhere from 8 to 16 hours a day at work, maybe more, so work plays a really big role in our weight loss efforts. Many people depend on regular paychecks to pay for their living expenses, but if your work environment is detrimental to your health, then you have to ask yourself if it is worth it. Or is there something else you could be doing, whether at your current job or a different one, to make your work environment healthier? Many corporations now have incentives for their employees to lose weight and stay healthier. Ask yourself, why haven't I participated in my employer's health program? Should I start a lunchtime walking group? Why don't I know where the stairs are located? What other lunch options are there other than our usual fast food or buffet places? Is there a good-intentioned co-worker who brings donuts every Monday? Perhaps the baked goods could stay in a less-tempting place in the building. If you spend this much time at work, shouldn't you take steps to make it more health-friendly? And if you don't take a stand, then who will?

4. *How did you spend your weekends prior to weight loss surgery?*

    Our "free time" is just that, free time. But how do you spend your free time? Do you waste it away by sleeping in until noon, then wonder why you can't sleep at night and why you feel sluggish come Monday morning? Or do you wake up before sunrise in order to finish all of the "chores" that you have to get done or promised others you'd get done? Either way, ask yourself if you are really participating in life and making your life the one you want, or are you letting life pass you by? Are you willing to change this? Personally, even though it is Super Bowl Sunday as I type this, and on most weekends I'm involved with family, patient, or professional activities, I leave the weekend often feeling that I could have accomplished more. But I guess this is better than feeling like I haven't accomplished anything at all. An accomplishment to me doesn't mean getting the laundry done, but teaching my daughter how to use the swing set, going with patients and staff to participate in a 5-K walk, or planting herbs. These are things I can't do on weeknights, and they make my weekend satisfying and memorable.

5. *How did you spend your family time? Name one activity you did together.*
    The important point is to realize that it is the FAMILY INTERACTION that is important. Did you spend your time making lasting memories or were you too busy in the kitchen, shuttling kids around, or shopping for more shoes to notice that you had missed out on those opportunities to make memories? What will you do differently moving forward? Many wonderful family memories involve doing something together, just family, outdoors.

6. *Name one charity for which you would like to volunteer and why.*
    I believe a lot in charity work. I have partnered my practice with many charities. My patients, staff, and our families participate in fundraisers and charity walks regularly. My two main partnerships are with the Snowdrop Foundation, which cares for children with cancer, and the Wounded Warrior Project, an international organization that helps American veterans who were wounded on the battlefield. I am on the board of D'Feet Breast Cancer, an organization that provides free mammograms and breast cancer care for impoverished women. We also volunteer for the Galveston Bay Foundation in trash cleanups and grass plantings in the bay area. But why do I point this out?

    I believe that it is critically important for your long-term weight maintenance to see the world from a broader perspective. Many people who struggle with their weight often become overwhelmingly self-focused. They may be filled with self-doubt and grow socially isolated. They may put themselves down or allow others to put them down, and the negative feelings this causes reinforces their poor habits. These poor habits, in turn, exacerbate the situation and it becomes very difficult for them to see beyond their own weight struggles. It can be tough to pull yourself out of this cycle, but it is key to your success. Often it can be achieved by forming meaningful connections with others and seeing the difficult challenges that others face and overcome.

    Thinking about the bigger picture will help put your weight struggles into perspective. Once they do not appear to be insurmountable, you'll see all the ways that you can empower yourself to become healthier and more vibrant. I believe deeply that donating your time and energy to a charity will help you to break free from that sense of isolation and fill your downtrodden spirit with renewed life and vigor! I honestly believe in that old saying: whatever you give you will receive back ten-fold. I have already seen it in my own life.

I immigrated to the United States as a little boy with just my father. We spent months in a refugee camp in Thailand, and then we were "sponsored" to come to America. We got off the plane in Houston with nothing but the clothes on our backs. We didn't even have a place to go. It was only through the generosity of the local government that we survived the night and by the generosity of a local church that we were able to set down roots. I've gotten to where I am today in my life, every step along the way, largely through the generosity of others, and I have not forgotten this. Years later, when I was in college at Rice University, I was living in a house off campus when I found my old papers that were given to me when I entered the Airport Authority. On those papers, the address of the people who had "sponsored" me was listed, and as it turned out, they lived on the same street where I currently was living! What were the odds? But they had moved away, so I never got to meet that family whose simple act of generosity changed my life forever. Isn't life funny that way?

What organization are you willing to give your time to? Whose life could you change? Money is always nice, but I've come to learn that most of these organizations just need your time, your free time. This is a win-win situation. They need your time, you've got time to give, and at the very least, you will get out of the house and get some physical activity. If you feel you don't have time, make it into a family activity or find something you can do during the lunch hour. There are so many organizations that need you, there is certainly one that will spark your interest and fit into the amount of time you have to give. Don't let this opportunity pass you by; at the end of the day you can feel that you have made the world a little of a better place.

7. *Write the first sentence of your journal entry for today.*
    This isn't the "Dear Diary" activity of adolescent girls, so don't be embarrassed. It is very important that you keep a journal. Write down what you did, how you were feeling when you did it, and why you think you did it. Your journal is the place where you can write down your thoughts and emotions and not worry about being judged. A simple spiral notebook will do just fine, but in today's world you can do this online. You can blog online, you can post online, you can join groups online. The important thing is you write it down. It may help you to understand the motivations that have led to your weight struggles and provide insight into how you can overcome them.

8. *Do you keep a food diary?*
    A questionnaire was given to those banded patients who had lost greater than 90 % of their excess weight. This questionnaire was hoping to find what these patients were doing differently from other less successful patients. The study found that these highly successful patients were doing one simple thing that the other group was not: they kept food diaries. While keeping a food diary might seem onerous to some, aren't the benefits worth it? A lot of patients willingly pay tens of thousands of dollars in cash for their surgeries. What would you be willing to pay to help you achieve that goal you are after? Would you pay $20 for a professionally bound food and exercise diary? How about paying $0.99 for a simple spiral notebook? Better than that, there are many online food diaries that will help you track your caloric intake for free. They can help you determine just how many calories a chicken breast or an ear of corn has. Just write down everything you eat, and seek out sites that help you gauge their nutritional value. You might like to try these online resources:

    *   *FitDay.com*—this free online resource gives you access to a weight loss journal, daily calorie counts, and nutritional information on thousands of foods.

    *   *www.bodybugg.com*—this is a small device that you wear on your arm that helps measure your daily caloric intake and expenditure.

- *FoodFit.com*—provides free expert information on healthy eating, healthy cooking, and fitness.

- *MoreFromMyBand.com*—this is my website. I write and send out my own weekly newsletters that are full of tips and insights from a surgeon's perspective.

9. *Name one thing that is different in your life since your surgery.*
   Give yourself some credit. Reflect on everything you've accomplished so far. Use this opportunity to set milestones in your weight loss journey, and I'm not just talking about the number on the scale, or the smaller clothing size, or the changes in your medication. Those are all good measures. But I think it is probably more important to acknowledge the other positive changes in your life. Are you a better mother because you have more energy to play with your children? Are you a better employee because you have more focus at work? Are you a better spouse because you are more emotionally available? Are you a better child because you help your family around the house and yard? Are you a better humanitarian because you donate your time to charities?

   If you can't think of anything, don't be embarrassed. Ask someone you love! They will give you an honest answer.

10. *What is one thing about your life that you will change right now?*
    It can be a big dream or a small step, but regardless of the immensity of the change, just go do it! Commit to it now. Whether your surgery took place last month, last year, or in the last decade, it was just the start of the journey. Now it is time to go live the rest of your life! Go make a difference. Be noticed. Leave a mark. Set an example. Be an inspiration to others. You can do this. You matter.

Notes

Section Two

The Maintenance Period

Getting the Lap-Band surgery is such an exciting step. You were likely highly motivated right after your surgery to be a healthier eater and more active person. The pounds probably dropped off quickly in those first weeks, and you were excited to be able to fit into smaller sizes. Coworkers, friends, and family were all impressed with the changes they saw and complimented your new lifestyle regularly. All of this positive attention gave you not only a morale boost, but also constant reinforcement. Sometimes it may have been hard learning how to eat, what to eat, and when to eat, but overall it was pretty easy to lose weight.

Now the surgery is in the distant past. Everyone has gotten used to the New You and nobody comments on how great you look except occasionally when you bump into an old acquaintance. You have deadlines at work, increasing family obligations, fun social activities planned, and a lot else going on. You need to focus on so many aspects of your life right now that leaving the car way across the parking lot and taking the stairs seems like a big waste of time and cooking a fresh meal will cut into your long list of things to do. Since you've shifted away from making your banded lifestyle your number one priority, your weight loss probably slowed or stopped. Perhaps you even put a few pounds back on.

If this has happened to you or if you want to avoid this scenario, then now is the time to read this next section. When asked what it is that I do for a living, most people would answer that I am a Lap-Band surgeon. I say, "No, I am a motivator of people." My number one job is to constantly motivate those around me, and that includes you reading this book. You need motivation to stick to your healthy choices and overcome your weight-loss "plateau." You can reach your happy weight, walk in a local 5K, get through the holidays without putting on pounds, or reach any of your other goals. You have the answers to your struggles, the trick is unlocking them. The aim of this section is to give you that motivational boost, to provide you with simple tips to get back on track, and to encourage you always to make your own health a priority.

Start by thinking about all you have accomplished in the past several months, both in terms of your health and the rest of your life. Give yourself proper credit for these accomplishments. And then resolve to accomplish even more.

Weight Loss Slow Down, a.k.a. Weight Loss Plateau

Answer these questions if your weight loss has slowed or if you have put weight back on. Come back to them as often as you need to stay on track.

1. List the three signs that indicate you might need a Lap-Band Adjustment.

   _____

   _____

   _____

   _____

2. Which one of the answers from question #1 do you rely on mostly?

   _____

   _____

3. Are you eating enough protein? How many grams of protein a day should you eat?

   _____

   _____

4. Could it be that you are drinking your daily calories?
   a. List any drinks you are consuming that contain calories and how frequently.

   _____

   _____

   _____

   _____

   b. What is wrong with diet drinks?

   _____

   _____

   _____

   _____

5. Could it be that you are not drinking enough water? How much water are you drinking a day? How much water should you be drinking a day?

_____

_____

_____

6. Could it be that you are not eating enough?
    a. How many times a day should you eat with the Lap-Band?

    _____

    b. What is the minimum number of calories you should consume to avoid metabolic slowdown?

    _____

    c. How can you combat a slow metabolism?

    _____

    _____

7. Are you consuming empty calories (calories without any nutritious value)? Any at all? Write down everything you have eaten since breakfast yesterday morning and evaluate your choices.

_____

_____

_____

Healthy Shopping Skills

1. Name three "impulse" items located in the store that you struggle with.

    _____

    _____

    _____

2. Identify one tactic to reduce "temptation" or "impulse" shopping.

    _____

    _____

3. Give an example of why buying in bulk can work against your weight management goals.

    _____

    _____

4. List three ways to save money and shop healthier in the grocery store.

    _____

    _____

    _____

5. Why are terms such as "sugar-free," "sugarless," "low fat" and "all-natural" misleading?

    _____

    _____

6. When reading labels, what should you focus on?

    _____

7. What would be a healthier choice for the food selections listed below?
    Whole Milk

    Butter

    Cheese

    White Rice

    White Bread

    Lunch Meat

8. List one unhealthy shopping habit that you have and how you will change it.
    _____
    _____

9. Will you commit to this change TODAY?
    _____

10. What is the First Rule of Lap-Band Eating?
    _____
    _____
    _____

Weight Loss Slow Down, a.k.a. Weight Loss Plateau

1. *List the three signs that indicate you might need a Lap-Band Adjustment.*
    The following diagram is adapted from Allergan, Inc. Most patients have
    seen a version of this chart at some point or another.

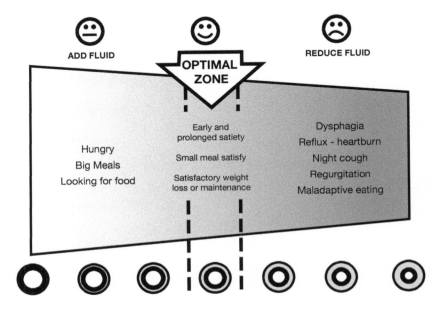

The three main signs that most people know are: you're hungry between
meals, you think you're eating too much, and you're not losing weight.

What do these signs mean when taken in context with everything else that
is happening in your life? By this I mean, for the fist sign, are you sure you
are really hungry? I teach my patients to try and figure out whether they
are really hungry or whether they are just feeling psychological hunger.
Real hunger manifests itself with measurable physical changes—decreased
blood sugar, weakness, sweating, jitteriness, dizziness, etc. Psychological
hunger does not come with these physical changes (even though your
stomach may still rumble), but rather is triggered by the thought, sight,
or familiar smell of food. This is often situational. For example, you
might develop cravings when a food commercial comes on while you're

watching your favorite TV show or you walk by a cookie stand. So if you feel hungry, make sure it is really hunger that you are feeling. Assess whether it is an appropriate time to be hungry and verify that you are not in a situation that could trigger psychological hunger. If you put yourself in a different situation – you turn off the TV and go outside or you move away from the smells of baking – you might find that you're not "hungry" a few minutes later.

A lot of my patients think they are eating too much (maybe this is because I scare them into thinking that they can only eat a little saucer full of food). After reviewing their meals, I am happy to point out to most of my patients that they are actually eating the right amount of food! It is just more than what they THOUGHT they should eat. Sometimes I point out that they should increase the texture of what they eat. Maybe they are scared to move away from fish and have been avoiding chicken or meat for fear that it would get stuck. "A meal" is something very different for a band patient. Sometimes this is very hard for patients to understand or recognize. A support group can help you determine whether you are eating appropriate band meals.

This leads us to the third familiar sign—not losing weight. While it is possible that you really are too loose and need an adjustment, you should also ask yourself if you are doing your part of the work. Cher Ewing, a banded life coach and friend, asks her clients, "Is the band failing you or are you failing your band?" Are you eating late at night? Are you eating empty calories? Have you not been back to see your surgeon in a while to see if everything is fine with your band? Have you not attended a support group in a long time? Are you not exercising? All of these things can result in weight gain even in a well-adjusted band patient.

In summary, while the three signs might indeed indicate that you need an adjustment, they might also instead indicate that there are some changes you need to make in your daily choices.

2. *Which one of the answers from question #1 do you rely on mostly?*
    Do you notice yourself relying on one signal more than the others? Why is that? The three should work in combination. I had one patient who, a week after her first adjustment, complained that she was hungry and thought the adjustment "didn't work" even though we explain to our patients that the average number of adjustments the first year is 4 or 5 and can vary between 2 and 10 or even more! After talking with her, it became apparent that she was stressed out about something. It was the one year anniversary of her father's passing. Eventually she said, "I don't even know why I am eating—I'm not even hungry when I do it..." which was the opposite of her original complaint. We hugged her really hard and encouraged her to come to support group because it was clear that she was failing her band. It was not a matter of her band failing her.

    If you are constantly asking your surgeon for a fill, then get too tight, then have to get all of the fluid removed, then get too tight again, at some point, you've got to ask yourself if it is something that you are doing that's the problem.

3. *Are you eating enough protein? How many grams of protein a day should you eat?*
    Remember the First Rule of Lap-Band Eating? "Yes, Dr. Vuong. Protein First." Great! But how much is enough? Most physicians recommend 50-60 grams per day of protein for the average person, but the necessary amount is probably even more for bandsters.

    "Yes, I know the number of grams, but how much should I EAT?" Putting the knowledge into practice is a struggle in itself. As a guideline, I recommend the "1-2-3 Rule for Protein." You should eat 1 ounce of protein for breakfast, 2 ounces for lunch, and 3 ounces for dinner. Ok, now how much is an ounce, you ask? A good approximation is that a deck of cards is about the size of 3 ounces of protein. One of those slim Motorola Razor cell phones is also about 3 ounces. Now you have a guide to go by. To get two ounces, just approximate a portion size about ⅔ the size of a deck of cards! Another easy trick is to remember that one boiled egg is about one ounce of protein. That should make breakfast a cinch!

4.   *Could it be that you are drinking your daily calories? List any drinks you are consuming that contain calories and how frequently. What is wrong with diet drinks?*

A Skinny Vanilla Latte Venti made with non-fat milk and no whipped cream from Starbucks still has 160 calories! I have a patient who used to drink 6 or 7 of these a day, even after she had her Lap-Band surgery, thinking she was making a good choice because they're made with non-fat milk and are called "skinny." Well, those 7 "skinny" drinks still added about 1000 calories a day to her diet! When she found out the REAL skinny on this drink, she quit her habit, and is now well on her way to weight loss success.

What about alcohol? Are you consuming empty calories with poor alcohol choices? If you don't remember the exact numbers on alcohol, please reread sections 1 and 2 for a refresher. A margarita can pack up to 600 calories! If you are at a party and absolutely must have a drink, wine is a lower-calorie option. A small glass still has about 100 calories, though, so don't overdo it.

"What about all of these new-fangled fancy-schmancy energy drinks, Dr. Vuong?" I say, if you need them for energy, then that should tell you that you are probably either 1) not getting proper nutrition, so your body is seeking that nourishment or 2) you've fallen for the multibillion dollar marketing hype. Most of these drinks pack a ton of calories. They take you on a sugar high only to let you crash a couple of hours later. Remember that calories are our body's source of energy, so anything that calls itself "energy," even if it has a picture of someone running uphill on it, is going to be full of calories.

"What is the problem with diet sodas?" you ask. Plenty. I discuss diet drinks more in the Resolutions chapter, but let me give you some things to think about here. One morning in my office, three new patients were sitting around the kitchen table, waiting on my dietitian to develop a 1200-Calorie meal plan with them, when I came in and poured myself a small cup of coffee. I put 2 sugar packets in my coffee. One of the patients, whose BMI was almost 55, said to me, "Dr. Vuong, you are setting a bad example for us. You are supposed to be demonstrating healthy choices."

"What's the problem?" I asked, knowing where this conversation was heading. My current BMI is 20. I like sugar in my coffee, but I only drink one cup a day.

She said, "Why are you putting sugar packets in your coffee? That's bad for you!"

I responded with, "I know where sugar comes from—sugar cane—but I don't know where the stuff in pink, blue, or yellow packets comes from."

The truth is, it's not any one item, like sugar or butter, which causes us to be obese. It's what we do on an everyday basis that matters. It doesn't make sense for you to order a Big Mac, French fries, milkshake—these three items add up to almost 2100 calories--and then think that you are making a good choice because you've also ordered a DIET coke. Diet sodas are often over-consumed because people think they are harmless. But they have no nutritious value and pour a lot of chemicals into your system. I would rather enjoy a small amount of real sugar than a lot of artificial sweeteners. And my body is healthier for it.

5. *Could it be that you are not drinking enough water? How much water are you drinking a day? How much water should you be drinking a day?*
    You are ⅔ water. And this ratio only gets higher the older and bigger you get. I know, there is just no justice in this world. But if this is how we were naturally created, then shouldn't we replenish our bodies with the most natural and best option—clean water? For those of you who say you don't like the "taste" of water, my answer is, you would love the "taste" of water if you were lost in the desert. You don't even need to be lost. Try this one experiment, if you don't believe me. Go for a walk or a hike where there are no convenience stores or drive-thru's around and bring only a bottle of water. Leave your water bottle at the starting point, do your walk, work up a sweat, and when you get back to the start, just try NOT to drink that water! You won't be able to; it will look too tempting. Do this exercise a couple of times and you'll be hooked on the "taste" of

water. Why do I put "taste" in quotation marks? Because water has no taste. If your water has a taste, it is not pure water.

How much water you should drink depends on your size and activity level, but it is usually around 8-10 eight-ounce glasses per day. Put very simply, you should drink water whenever you are thirsty to ensure you are drinking enough of it. Start replacing one of your non-water drinks per day with water, and every week replace another until all of your drinks are water. Of course, there will be some exceptions, but drinking water should be the main way you quench your thirst.

6. *Could it be that you are not eating enough? How many times a day should you eat with the Lap-Band? What is the minimum number of calories you should consume to avoid metabolic slowdown? How can you combat a slow metabolism?*

    We teach our patients to eat 3 meals a day, plus a snack if you are diabetic or are truly hungry between meals. Some clinics don't think banded patients can eat in the mornings because the band is "tighter" in the mornings. While I believe that it is probably harder to eat in the mornings due to dry mucus that has accumulated during the night, this is no excuse not to eat. You have to eat something, if for nothing more than the caloric intake. We teach our patients to eat breakfast and to think about breakfast in a different way than Denny's restaurant would like. Breakfast should be something as simple as an egg or a protein drink plus a third of a banana.

If you are hungry between meals, do not "tough it out" until the next meal time. This is because you just can't physically eat enough at one sitting to make up for that hunger craving. This will leave you very frustrated. Remember my patient who used to work all day, skip meals, and be ravenous when she got home? Don't fall into that cycle. Have the snack, and your next meal will be an appropriately-sized Lap-Band meal. Make sense? Of course, by snack, I mean a good snack—not candy, twinkies, cookies, chips, or anything else that can cause your blood sugar to spike and crash. This is not a Free Pass to splurge. Have the rest of your breakfast banana, for example.

Any very low caloric diet (VLCD) requires monitoring by a physician. These are typically meal replacement diets where the caloric intake is less than 1000 calories per day. Let me repeat myself: these absolutely have to be monitored by a physician. An example of such a program is Optifast 800 Meal replacement Program, which takes patients down to 800 calories a day. The physician should perform regular, routine lab work to check your blood chemistries and your kidney and liver functions.

The medical field is pretty sure now that when caloric intake drops down to around 1100-1200 calories per day, human metabolism will slow down. This is a natural, evolutionary response. Think back to the Caveman again. When humans had to scavenge for food that was not always readily available, our bodies became very efficient at storing energy in the form of fat to tide us through times when we might not be able to eat much for a few days. When food became scarce, our metabolism would slow down in order to conserve energy, at least until food became plentiful again. Typically your body will go into this energy-conserving mode if you drop your caloric intake to around 1100-1200 calories per day. Since a well-adjusted Lap-Band should take you down to around this amount, your body will want to go into hibernation mode. Your job is to keep this from happening. How do you do this, you ask?

With two simple steps:
- Make sure you are getting the best nutrition you can. This means eating real food, avoiding empty calories, preparing fresh meals, and buying organic foods whenever possible. This will give your body all of the micronutrients and building blocks it needs to perform its normal daily chemical reactions that keep us feeling good.

- Exercise. This will keep your metabolism going by releasing natural hormones that control our "fight or flight" response. Ever heard of a "runner's high?" Sometimes getting started with an exercise routine is tough, but think back about how great you felt after a work out—not just the feeling of accomplishing something, but how energized and alert you were. That's a natural response. It had very little to do with your expensive gym equipment, your personal trainer with rock hard abs, or your perfectly set iPod tunes. It had everything to do with what a wonderful machine the human body is.

Have you ever heard, "The last 20 pounds are the hardest to lose"? Wonder why this is? My guess is that people who complain about this would benefit from following the steps outlined above. The last twenty pounds are really the same as the first twenty, but your body percentages are different. You need to keep making the healthiest choices possible all along the way.

7. *Are you consuming empty calories (calories without any nutritious value)? Any at all? Write down everything you have eaten since breakfast yesterday morning and evaluate your choices.*
    If you are not losing weight, and especially if you are GAINING weight, then you are consuming too many empty calories—pure and simple.

If you want long-term weight-loss success, then you really must keep a food diary. There are no excuses when you keep a food diary—the evidence is right there in front of you. Our minds subconsciously try to ameliorate our feelings to avoid hurting us psychologically, and sometimes this can undermine our weight-loss efforts. Remember that time you were going to eat just one girl scout cookie, and before you knew it, the whole box was gone, and you didn't even realize it? Why was that? How did that happen? If you know that you will be accountable for every cookie, it's not as easy to keep eating. When you know that you will have to count up all the empty slots in that cookie box and then calculate how many calories that equaled and write it in your food diary, you'll find yourself able to stop after one or two, or maybe you won't even open the box at all.

We have evidence that people who have excellent and lasting weight loss are the ones who keep food diaries. They are dedicated to writing down not only the calories they consume, but also the activities they do, AND all of the emotions they were feeling at the time of eating or exercising. Keeping a food journal is like anything else—it's a little difficult to get started, but once you get going, it just becomes second nature. That little extra effort is definitely worth saying goodbye to those pounds – forever.

Notes

Healthy Shopping Skills

1. *Name three "impulse" items located in the store that you struggle with.*

   Has this ever happened to you? You say you are just going to make a quick trip to the grocery store for some toilet paper, or milk, or whatever little item you need. You frantically run through the store to get the item you need so you can make it back home in time for American Idol, but wait a minute! The bag of chips or your favorite cookies or the diet coke is on sale, or if you buy one you'll get the second one free—so you've got to buy it, right? It's just too good of a deal! And why is that sale item always at the end of the isle so that in your rush to turn the corner, you always happen to run into it? That store manager should really do a better job of placing his sale items in a proper place so that shoppers who are in a hurry, like you, aren't slowed down when you run into them. You would stop to give him this suggestion, if you weren't already so late. When you're walking to your car, instead of just a gallon of milk, you notice you have a whole bag of stuff!

   Impulse buying can be significant like this or simply buying a candy bar while you're waiting in line or grabbing a Starbucks (again, how convenient they are now often located inside the grocery store) to drink while you shop.

   It is really imperative that you learn all of the stocking tricks that grocery stores use to get you to buy more. These are time-tested and proven methods that they employ on you! Ever wonder why the cheap, individually wrapped, easy-to-pick-up gum, candy, batteries, etc. are at the check out line? Ever notice that the sugary cereals are at eye-level and all of the healthy stuff is up high or down low or even in an entirely different section of the store? Did you know that producers pay more money to have grocery chains stock their items in these prime locations? It is not just by coincidence that you enter a store only wanting to buy some milk and leave with a bag full of treats.

2. *Identify one tactic to reduce "temptation" or "impulse" shopping.*

    You will find endless lists available on the internet and web forums on this topic. It seems like every New Year's there's always a story on this topic adapted to the current atmosphere. This year with the economic downturn, it seemed like I saw several articles on "How to shop on a budget without ruining your diet," or something to that effect. The tips are usually a rehash of the same old stuff. But in case you've never seen one, here are some tips to help you get started:

    *   Don't shop when you're hungry.
    *   Make a list--know what you need and buy only what you need.
    *   Walk the perimeter of the store where the fresh produce, meats, and fish are.
    *   Look up and down (tempting items are placed at eye level and ends of the aisles).
    *   Avoid interior aisles all together.
    *   If possible, don't shop with young kids.
    *   If you have to bring the kids, then make shopping a learning experience. Point out the names of the fresh produce, and explain where they came from. That's a good way to practice geography since most stores sell produce that comes from all over the world. Use math by showing them how to weigh the items and figure out the cost. Teach them proper serving sizes in order to plan meals.

3. *Give an example of why buying in bulk can work against your weight management goals.*

    I have many friends who swear by the savings found in big warehouse stores like Sam's or Costco, but unless you own a small business, I don't really understand the benefits of shopping at one of these stores. Ask yourself, "Do I really need all of the extra food lying around?" If it is in your home, it will be readily available, and most of the bulk items are "snack foods," not ingredients that can be used to cook healthy meals. What I have found when perusing these stores is that most of the items have a shelf-life, which means they are processed and not what I consider to be real food. While yes, some have meats and seafood, most of it is not good quality meat and most of the seafood is frozen. Much of the fruit or produce is not any cheaper than that in the regular stores overall. Next time you are there, just take a peak at what is in other peoples' carts. Ask yourself, "Is this REAL food that I am providing for my family?"

As I've mentioned before, Hurricane Ike came through my area this past fall 2008 and devastated lots of homes. My neighborhood had 7 feet of water in most places, including inside my home. We were without power for almost one month. Many people came back to tons of rotten and spoiled foods in their freezers and refrigerators. The stench was unbearable the first few days after the hurricane. Many people had to throw out multiple freezers full of bad food, spoiled hunting meat, and rotten fish from multiple fishing trips. And as I drove around, I asked myself, why did these people need so much food? Especially frozen food? Did they know something that I did not? Were they hoarding food for a reason? The last problem we have in this country is a shortage of available food.

There is also another problem with having large quantities of food lying around. Studies have shown that we will eat whatever serving size is placed in front of us. So if you buy a big jug or container of something, it will most likely be consumed AND in the same amount of time as a smaller jug or container of the same item. For example, if you buy a jumbo container of pretzels, most likely they will be eaten in the same amount of time that it would have taken to eat a small bag. In other words, if you are buying a big supply of food thinking it will last longer or that it will somehow save you time by decreasing your trips to the store, you're fooling yourself. This is true for anything—chips, cookies, soda bottles, etc. Probably not fresh fruit though—that will probably spoil. Why would your kids choose to eat fresh fruit when there is a huge bag of cookies right next to it?

So next time, consider this. Is the money you're saving (and even that point is debatable) really worth the harm you are doing to your body or to your family?

4. *List three ways to save money and shop healthier in the grocery store.*
    Everyone thinks I'm crazy, but I shop for one meal at a time. If I am feeling particularly adventurous that day, I might shop for two meals like dinner that night and brunch the next day. Even with my hectic schedule, I still find time to cook 4 or 5 dinners every week for my family. People always ask me how I find time. I respond, "How do you NOT have time?" I just make it a priority. It is important to me to provide my family with fresh, healthy meals as frequently as possible. This is a way that I show them my love. And I don't mean cooking them deep-fried greasy foods in huge proportions that bust open their belts, either. That's not love in my opinion; that is killing them slowly with food. I don't have snacks lying around, either—if I shop every day, I don't need "handy (prepackaged) snacks," because I always have fresh food available. But if you are going to be a frequent flyer at the grocery store, there are some things you need to know.

- **Avoid marketing gimmicks**, like "New and Improved," "Even Cheesier," "30% more FREE," "Buy 2 Get 1 Free" (unless there are bargains on nonperishable items, like toilet paper, of course). There will always be something on sale or something improved, and it is more economical over all to just stick to what you need.

- **Buy just what you need for your meals**. If you are buying fresh, then you should only be shopping around the perimeter of the store. A lot of patients are surprised by how much money they save when they pass on the frozen meals, the extra snacks, and the unnecessary impulse buys.

- **Buy organic foods**. I know what you are thinking because I thought the same thing initially. Why should I pay $2.99/lb for organic broccoli when the regular broccoli is only $1.99/lb? (You can substitute whatever item.) Organic foods can be 2, 3, or 4 times as expensive as the conventional variety. Today I bought organic chicken breast for $8.99/lb when the regular chicken breast next to it was only $4.99/lb. But the difference in nutritional value for certain vitamins and minerals can be 10, 100, or even 1000 times greater in organic foods, easily justifying their higher price. And that doesn't even take into account all the chemicals that are avoided. So I just decided that I am worth that extra dollar or two for my organic broccoli. More importantly, I decided that my family is worth it. If you forgo that package of cookies, you'll be able to buy organic and still save some money.

- **Avoid items with a shelf-life**. These foods are highly processed and injected with preservatives and chemicals that you just don't need.

5. *Why are terms such as "sugar-free," "sugarless," "low fat," and "all-natural" misleading?*
   These labels are mostly marketing ploys and don't have any real meaning behind them. Most of the time, these labels don't address the actual nutritional value of food. Also if these "foods" have packages that allow the manufacturers to place the labels, then they are probably processed and prepackaged and therefore are not real foods that you need to be eating.

   "All-natural," "hormone-free," and such have various meanings but none of them carry as much weight as "organic." A chicken that is raised in a small and filthy coop, injected with antibiotics, and fed "food" that no chicken has business eating can be labeled "all-natural." What is "natural" after all? There is no regulation on what counts as natural, and anyone can apply that and other similar terms to their products. However, the label "USDA-certified organic" means that the chicken was raised in a clean environment, fed USDA-certified organic feed, not injected with antibiotics, treated humanely, and raised according to a number of other standards, including fair labor laws. No sewage sludge can be used as a fertilizer for organic produce, no food can be irradiated or bioengineered, and growing methods have to be environmentally sustainable or "green." Furthermore, government officials have checked the facility on a regular basis to ensure that it meets these criteria. There are very few cases of fraudulent organic labeling, because not only does the government monitor this label, but other organic farmers monitor it. They want consumers to feel secure that their products are better than the non-organic versions so that they can charge more for them. Consumer advocacy groups also verify that the organic labeling is justified. There is a lot of internal regulation taking place that makes that organic seal significant. "Organic," therefore, is the only food claim I would hang my hat on.

6. *When reading labels, what should you focus on?*
    This is somewhat of a trick question. If the food has a nutrition label, then you probably shouldn't eat it or at least not eat it on a regular basis. Remember it's the everyday things we do that matter. So if every night before bed you settle down for your bedtime snack, then the fact that it has X,Y,Z nutrition amounts on its food label is less important than the fact that you are eating it every night before bed. You see my point? And I don't care if it says "Sugar-Free," "Fat-Free," "Made with real fruit," etc. on the label. If you eat real food regularly and labeled food sparingly, you'll be doing pretty well.

    If you insist on reading food labels then here are the items you should focus on:

    *   Look at the number of calories, but also note the serving size — a single cookie could in fact be labeled as 2 servings, so you would need to double the calorie and fat quantities if you expect to eat the whole cookie.
    *   Be careful of the salt and fat content.
    *   And remember the First Rule? Note the protein content.

7. *What would be a healthier choice for the food selections listed below?*
    *   Whole Milk—soy milk is best. Remember this the next morning you are thirsty: an 8oz glass of whole milk has the equivalent of a pat of butter in it.

    *   Butter—olive oil is better, but at least I know where butter comes from. I don't know what margarine is, so definitely avoid margarine and lard.

- Cheese—buy REAL cheese, the stuff from the deli that costs $10 for an 8 oz block. Use it to augment your meal (like a serving of fruit and cheese as an appetizer), not as the main ingredient in your dish, like lasagna or mac-and-cheese.

- White Rice—brown rice is better, or at least rice without the "flavorings." Couscous, quinoa, and simple polenta are even better choices because they contain more nutrients and fiber.

- White Bread—no bread is best, but wheat bread or multi-grain bread is better. Be careful, though, some "wheat" breads are merely white breads with food coloring. Choose breads with a fiber content of at least 3 grams per slice.

- Lunch Meat—lunch meats are filled with preservatives and flavorings, so buy real cooked meats, like roast chicken.

8. *List one unhealthy shopping habit that you have and how you will change it.*
This is a personal answer, but we all could do better. Take me as an example. For special occasions and parties, I used to buy a chocolate mousse pie from the bakery. I liked it so much, one weekday I bought it for dessert for after dinner. My family and I ate pieces of it for a couple of days and were happy. I then started trying the different pies and cakes the bakery had to offer, and before I knew it, I bought dessert on almost every shopping trip. It wasn't until my partner started complaining about her figure that I made the connection—and I do this for a living! Now we save the pies for very special occasions and eat fresh fruit after dinner every night.

You probably know what you are doing wrong in the shopping department. Are you buying too many prepackaged foods, sweets, sodas, chips, artificially-flavored foods, or impulse treats in too great of a quantity? Are you not buying enough fresh fruits and vegetables, real meats, or other real foods that spoil?

Here is an easy tip: add one good item to your cart now BEFORE you start taking away a bad item. Do this regularly and before you know it, your cart will be full of MOSTLY good items.

9. *Will you commit to this change TODAY?*

   Why wait any longer? Make changes that matter now. Quit fretting about it. Quit worrying about what your family will think or what your kids will say. Quit worrying about what your friends will do or your coworkers will mention. None of it matters. Take action today. Do something for yourself.

10. *What is the First Rule of Lap-Band Eating?*

    Are you starting to understand why the First Rule is so important? Everything you do as a banded patient will go back to it. Protein First. That means go pick up your protein first, then your fruits and veggies, then your essential non-perishables, and then if you have any money left, you can maybe get a nonessential item. If you are preparing fresh meals with a focus on good protein, then it only makes sense that you follow this shopping order. This is how I shop. I always shop with a meal in mind, and if I am not sure whether the store is going to have the key meat ingredient, like lamb chops or whole fish, then I go to the meat and fish department first and adjust my meal plan if necessary. Then I plan my side dishes. Then I pick up the paper towels, trash bags, or soap or whatever, then I pay for my items and leave the store. Shopping this way does not take long, and I can always use the express lane.

Notes

Holiday Eating Tips

Happy holidays – whether it's the 4th of July, Thanksgiving, or your yearly cruise! Congratulations for wanting to maintain healthy eating strategies during this time. Below are some good rules for anyone who wants to maintain their weight during the holidays. After these, I add some extra tips specifically for Lap-Band patients.

1. **Don't Start a Diet**

    Dieting during the holidays or on a vacation almost never works. It will not only frustrate you but also detract from the real reason for the holidays— to celebrate family bonds, enjoy yourself and the company of others, and make new and lasting memories. Instead, make it a goal to **just maintain your weight**. This will allow you to enjoy the holidays or vacation while remaining mindful of your health.

2. **Eat a Light Snack Before You Go**

    If you are going to a party, **eat ahead of time**. Saving "room" for all the great food is nothing but a recipe for disaster. If you arrive at a party hungry, chances are you will choose calorie-dense foods. (This is a natural, biologic response.) Instead, try eating enough healthy food beforehand so that you're satisfied before you arrive. You'll have much more self-control around those tempting party treats. And you will have given your body the nutrients it needs (no, it does not need anything found in a slice of pie).

3. **Give Up the "I've Already Blown It" Mentality**

    Have you ever said, "I've already ruined my diet, so it doesn't matter what I eat now?" There are times when we all make poor food choices, but that doesn't mean you have to throw in the towel! Step back from the situation, reassess, acknowledge the choice you made, then move forward with a renewed commitment to do better. It's never too late to stop, and it's nothing to be ashamed about. Keep in mind that weight is based on calories consumed and calories expended, so every decision you make matters. Everyone overeats sometimes, but your goal is to **contain the**

damage already done, not give up. Keeping a food diary will keep you accountable for all those calories that might seem as though they don't count because you eat them after you've already splurged. But stopping a splurge before you order a second margarita is far better than going ahead with a second, third, and fourth!

4. **Plan Ahead**

    Think about what you are going to eat when you get to a party or family gathering. Even go so far as to **write down what you will eat**. This will empower you to take control of the situation, and empowerment is the key to success in all things, not just weight loss. It will help you to remain conscious of your choices and to avoid slipping into mindless eating patterns. You'll feel even more accountable if you go back to your list and write down what you actually did eat and compare your choices with your plan.

5. **Know Who the "Saboteurs" Are**

    Every family has someone who tries, whether deliberately or not, to sabotage others' weight loss efforts. They are "diet killers or diet destroyers." **Have a response ready** for these people who try to tempt you with sweets and treats. The truth usually works well, like "I am trying to make healthier choices." But sometimes the saboteur will still push that fried chicken in front of you. Here are a few lines that my patients have told me that are really hard for any saboteur not to heed: "I have blood work for my (physical, annual, etc.) on Monday, and my doctor told me that (tempting item) could ruin the results;" "I have a toothache right now;" "I was told that food type would interfere with some medication I am taking;" "My husband and I have a tradition of sharing dessert alone with each other every holiday, so I am saving up for that later tonight, but thanks anyway!"

6. **Enlist an Army of More Than One**

    Going at it by yourself can be lonely, so **get the support of your friends and family**. Talk openly about the healthy changes you're making and try to encourage them to do the same. I always encourage my banded patients to tell their friends and family about their surgery because family get-togethers are very important in our society. Ultimately the responsibility is yours but you'll be much more successful in the long run if everyone's on the same page and tries to help you achieve your goals.

7. **"I'll Be Good Tomorrow" Doesn't Work**

Don't fool yourself into thinking that consuming fewer calories the day after the holiday or week after the vacation will work. An excessive dinner or party can undo a lot of treadmill walking. I recommend exercising a little every day for the entire week before the party. Don't even try telling yourself that you'll make it up the day after the party, unless you can safely commit to six hours at the gym! If you're going on a cruise, sign up for an activity that gets you walking or exercising every day. Nearly every boat and hotel has a gym these days, or physical outings, or a map of local walking trails. Keep in mind that walking one mile burns 100 calories for 130 pounds. If you weigh 260 pounds, you will burn 200 calories for each mile you walk. That means walking 3 miles to burn off just one margarita! Because margaritas come with chips and dip usually, expect to need another three-mile walk. And if you add a slice of apple pie, add a third walk. Walking nine miles takes a lot of time, but consuming those treats takes just a few minutes. That's why a full week of extra exercise is needed to make up for one evening of decadence.

8. **Allow Yourself a Taste of Your "Favorite"**

Did you know the chemical triggers that evoke our desires for a certain food are satisfied within the first 2 or 3 bites? So if (like one of my patients) key lime pie is your favorite, then **allow yourself 2 or 3 bites**. Understand the choice you are making and leave the guilt at home, but stick to just a small taste (each bite may contain 50 calories or more). Since it may be hard to push away the rest of the slice, make sure your initial portion is quite small. Then you can safely clean your plate! Or share one dessert with 3 friends.

9. **Beware of the Booze**

Besides lowering your inhibitions so that you're more likely to make poor choices, margaritas and other **sugary mixed drinks can pack around 600 calories**. Plus, drinks are often served with high-calorie snacks. (See chapters one and two for more information on alcohol.) If you really want to have that margarita Saturday night, plan for it by walking 30 minutes a day Monday through Friday. Depending on how fast you walk and on your size, that's about how much walking it takes to burn off a single margarita (see #7)! That should make that second round a lot less tempting. Definitely do not think that forgoing a nutritious dinner will cancel out the calories in the margarita, either. If you're hungry, and then you start drinking, you will be far more likely to eat high-fat and high-calorie foods.

10. **Think about Feeling Full**

It takes 20-25 minutes for chemicals from your stomach to reach your brain and signal satiety. So **don't wolf down your food** like it's a race to the finish. Instead slow down, taste your food, and enjoy your company like a leisurely Sunday drive through the countryside. A good trick is to make sure to put your fork down between every bite. If you do this, not only will you learn to recognize when you're full, it will probably take you longer than others to get through your meal so you won't have time for a second helping.

In addition to the above, the following are good reminders for banded patients.

11. **Remember the First Rule**

What is the First Rule of Lap-Band Eating? Protein First! That means pass on the chips and dips, appetizers, finger foods, etc, and focus on good protein, like fish, chicken, or turkey. Once you have eaten your protein, then see if you are still hungry and perhaps have a vegetable side dish.

12. **No Band Likes a Sloppy Drunk**

Excessive alcohol intake is one of the worst enemies of social eating for banded patients. Besides the extra calories, the loss of inhibition will make it harder to listen to your band signals, like when to stop eating, remembering to take small bites, and chewing your food well. Eat your protein first, wait 30 minutes, then consume your alcoholic beverages if you must. But make sure to plan your alcohol consumption carefully to avoid taking in too many extra calories.

13. Salad is NEVER a Good Choice

Protein first, protein first, protein first. I can't say it enough. Despite its reputation as a health food, salad is often low in nutrition and the roughage can be tough to digest—that can make for an embarrassing social situation. Also, many salad dressings are dense in calories and fat, so salad is not always a healthy option.

Enjoy the holidays or vacation, focus on friends and family, fit in some time for walking or other exercise, and make smart food choices whenever you can!

Notes

Top 10 Realistic Resolutions That Will Make a Difference

We all do it every year – we make New Year's resolutions that we really mean to keep, we feel so motivated to follow through, and then we abandon them a few days or, if we're lucky, a few weeks later. The problem of why we can't stick to our resolutions is often because our goals are too vague ("I will lose weight," "I will eat healthier," or "I will exercise," for example). Other resolutions are too unrealistic ("I will lose 50 pounds by Valentine's," "I will cut out all junk food"). Without a lot of support, it is hard to stick to the best of intentions when those around us have significantly different ideas and unwittingly sabotage our resolutions to become healthier, fitter, and ultimately happier.

My Top 10 Resolutions That Will Make A Difference list is concrete and manageable. You will not have to wake up two hours earlier every day to train for an Ironman competition or nibble on nothing but rabbit food. You can fit these healthy changes into your current lifestyle and not cause misery to yourself and those around you by trying to do too much too soon.

If you are reading this in July, there's no need to wait six months to make these resolutions. They work just as well in the summer as they do in the winter. Today, no matter the date, is the first day of the rest of your life, so resolve to make it a healthier one!

10. **Drink water**—We are made up of two-thirds water. Why not replenish and nourish our bodies with the Real Stuff? If people tell me "I don't like the taste of water," I tell them that is just an excuse because water has no taste (unless it's coming from a rusty pipe, of course!). If people ask me for suggestions on the best "flavored water," I ask them why they feel the need for the extra chemicals. For me the best flavored water is purified water with a squeeze of lemon. You can also chill water with cucumber slices for a refreshing and chemical-free drink. Drinking more water will also help retrain your body not to expect flavor to flow into it throughout the day. Drinking water will quickly become second nature, because it's what our bodies were designed to do.

9. **Give up Diet Sodas**—"What's wrong with diet sodas? They don't have any calories!" I hear this all of the time from patients. First, even with zero calories, do you really need all of the artificial chemicals in your body? Read the ingredients and you'll see that the diet soda does not sound like a food at all, but rather like a chemistry experiment. Secondly, studies suggest that diet sodas are more often consumed by overweight people than normal weight people—what does that tell us? Research shows that exposure to the artificial sweeteners in diet sodas increases our taste preference for sweeter foods. This means that if you drink diet sodas, you make it harder on yourself to give up sweets because your taste buds now need even sweeter foods to satisfy them!

8. **Give up all bread (and pasta)**—This is a simpler way of saying, "Eliminate all highly processed white flour from your diet." When people ask me what they can do to lose weight other than giving up sweets and sodas, I tell them, "It's simple; just give up bread in all of its forms." This means don't eat breadsticks, don't sop up gravy with the biscuit, don't eat the hamburger or hot dog bun, don't eat the pizza crust, don't order the "bottomless pasta dish." No tortilla chips, no nachos, no toast. You name it—if it comes from processed flour, avoid it like the plague. Our society presents us with white-flour-based "extra" items throughout the day so it is easy to mindlessly consume hundreds of calories without recognizing that we've actually eaten.

7. **Eat a variety of color**—Unfortunately, when you look at the plate of a typical overweight person, you will notice the predominance of one color—yellow, usually in various shades, like beige or tan. In other words, the color of FAT. Isn't it ironic that while many people struggle with their weight, the food they eat is the color of the substance they are trying to avoid? Start by adding one item of food that has a different color, like broccoli, and then go from there. But don't fool yourself. If you cover your broccoli with cheese sauce, you've just turned your green food back into (you guessed it) yellow goo! Eating a variety of colors is also a good way to ensure that you are getting better nutrition and consuming fewer calories because you will be eating more fresh produce.

6. **Use your cell phone to take a picture of everything you eat—** This is a tip from Dr. Terry Simpson from Arizona. Take a picture of everything you eat and drink throughout the day. At the end of the day, print out your photos and arrange them in front of you on the table. Now, there is no way to fool yourself about what you have (or have not) eaten! After you do this for a few days, you may find that there are certain times you eat more (during late-night television) or places that encourage you to overindulge (perhaps a certain restaurant). Knowing what your triggers are will help you plan to avoid them. Whenever you feel you've reached a weight-loss plateau, try doing this for a few days so that you can honestly assess what choices you are making. This tip works well with #7: aim to have a multicolored photo collection at the end of the day!

5. **Read one book on healthier living, like Fast Food Nation by Eric Schlosser or What to Eat by Marion Nestle—**It's like what G.I.Joe said at the end of every cartoon: "Now you know, and KNOWING is half the battle!" It is crucial to become more informed about nutrition—just be sure to seek real information, not fad diets or scams or cheats. Anything that claims it will revolutionize your life, create a whole new you, allow you to lose half your body size in a couple of months, or anything else that sounds far-fetched is not the kind of reliable, scientific, well-researched information that will help you in the long-run. Don't rely on the materials in the check-out aisle of the grocery store. Find a well-researched book by someone with good credentials.

4. **Give up on diets—**Why "Die-it" when you can "Live-it"? Where has dieting gotten you all of these years? It's time to do something different. Start by rethinking yourself and your self-worth. Understand what a valuable person you are and recognize how you deserve a better life! How much has the world missed out on because you are not participating in life? It's time for you to get back out there and Live It! A diet is a short-term quick fix that will ultimately fail you; instead ensure you are taking proactive steps to live the life you want.

3. **Make small changes that add up**—It doesn't make any sense to write a lofty goal like "I want to win the Boston Marathon" when you don't even own a pair of running shoes. It's the small changes that we can stick to (not the grand schemes) that are sustainable, and it's these small changes that will eventually add up to the big change in your health that you are after. So start small and build up momentum. In case you can't think of any, here are a few to get you started: take the stairs instead of the elevator, make time for 3 ten-minute walks that add up to your 30-minutes-a-day workout, use the next smaller sized plates (not the smallest) at meals, add one new good food to your regular shopping list BEFORE you take away an old bad food, or substitute one soda or diet soda a day for pure water. Once your small changes become second nature, add another and then another. Do this throughout the year and you'll have adopted a much healthier lifestyle without having to overhaul your entire existence.

2. **Think about how what you consume makes you feel**—I know this sounds all New Age Touchy-Feely and such, but it is just true. You have to understand what role food is playing in your life, how it is comforting, why it helps you to relax, what pain it is relieving, and what issue it is covering up that you are not wanting to face. This is often the most frightening step to becoming healthier—baring your soul so that you can examine it, for all of its faults, but also for all of its wonders! Then seek more effective ways to feel better and relax that won't sabotage your health. Reach out to friends, enjoy evening walks, and find other strategies to get the emotional benefits you may have been looking for in food.

1. **Write down your goals**—This is the key to success in any and all endeavors, not just weight loss. Your goals and desires take on a whole new life and meaning when you commit them to paper. Remember to put your List of Goals some place where you can read it every day, so that they will take hold in your subconscious. Be specific ("I will walk for 30 minutes 3 days per week" instead of "I will exercise") and be true to who you are (if you hate going to the gym, do not waste money on a new gym membership.)

Of course, reading through the resolutions is the easy part, but reading is not the most important step. The most important step is to DO! These should not be difficult to fit into your daily life. Select a few or all of these resolutions and slowly incorporate them into your routine. And never, ever feel that if one day you eat a plate of pasta with diet soda and then go through a big chocolate bar while lying on the couch that you have failed! Doing it once is not an excuse to do it again. Everybody falls off the wagon sometimes. The important question is "What am I going to do from this point forward?"

It's the patterns of behavior that affect our health the most. If on most days you drink water, walk for 30 minutes, and eat a variety of fresh fruits and vegetables, but occasionally slip up, you will be much healthier than someone who goes to the gym for two hours and avoids all fat but only keeps it up for a week.

Here's to a healthy and prosperous New Year (even in July).

Notes

Final Thoughts

Although you've reached the end of this book, you have certainly not reached the end of the road. My hope is that this book has demonstrated that you can reach your goals and, more importantly, that you can always set new ones. Leading and maintaining a healthy lifestyle is an on-going process, and there is always room for improvement.

One of the most effective ways to keep on track is to continually educate yourself in the many facets of health. Now that you've finished this book, perhaps you might be interested in researching food safety, walking programs, local volunteering activities, nutrition, or anything else that has piqued your interest.

As you continue on your journey, keep these tips in mind. Over time, they will become automatic habits:

- **Avoid the white carbs**, meaning foods made with processed white flour like white bread, white pasta, etc. Not only do these cause your blood sugar to spike and then plummet, they offer little nutrition and are often added as calorie-dense "extras" to meals.

- **Exercise a little every day**. If you know you have a hectic day ahead of you, set your alarm a little earlier to walk around the neighborhood or fit in three 10-minute walks or take several flights of stairs as you go about your tasks. Whenever you can, aim to do more continuous exercise of a higher intensity. (And no, "whenever" does not mean once a year, but about three times per week or more.)

- **Eat like a caveman**. Remember, this means avoid processed and pre-packaged foods. Eat fresh, cook your own meals, and fill your plate with protein and vegetables.

- **Fill your pouch with the most nutritious food you can**. Because you will be taking in fewer calories than before, make sure they count. Do not drink your calories except on very special occasions.

- **What's the First Rule of Lap-Band Eating**? That's right, Protein First!

- **Be happy**. My goal for my patients is to have them love food again, love themselves, and take pride in their accomplishments. If you slip up, take stock of all you have accomplished and set reasonable goals on what you can expect to do today (a 20-minute lunchtime walk? A home-cooked dinner? Healthy lunch choices?). It's all the little choices we make hundreds of times each day that determine whether or not we will succeed.

- **Remember that you are worth it**. Focus on surrounding yourself with positive reinforcement and people who want to help you succeed. Your health is vital and should never take a backseat to all your other obligations. Go participate in life and show the WORLD that you are WORTH it!

Remember to come back to your answers in this book every few months. They will help you gauge how far you've come. You might also want to join a local support group or sign up for my support group DVDs, available at MoreFromMyBand.com. You can also send me a note or write on my wall on Facebook. Just search for Dr. V's Gastric Band Group, then add me as a friend. Remember, the answer lies within you. Now go out and make a difference in the world!

RESOURCES *

Awesome Support Websites

- *www.MoreFromMyBand.com*
  My personal website with my personal weekly newsletters and information on my FREE Lap-Band Giveaway.

- *www.WeightLossSurgeryChannel.com*
  The only internet news channel devoted solely to helping weight loss surgery patients. It has regular shows, broadcasts, and an online forum. Check them out, you'll be hooked.

- *www.LapbandTalk.com*
  A huge online community for banded patients only. I post here regularly also.

- *www.BandedTogether.net*
  Life Coach Cher Ewing, herself a banded patient, sends out a weekly informative newsletter. We often coordinate events together, so be watching for upcoming announcements.

- *www.lapband.com*
  The official site of Allergan, the makers of the Lap-Band.

- *www.REALIZEband.com*
  Ethicon's support website for their Realize band, Lap-Band's only U.S. competitor.

- *www.TrueResults.com*
  One of the largest collective experiences with the Lap-Band.

- *www.TexasCitySurgical.com*
  Learn more about my practice.

- *Dr.V's Gastric Band Group on Facebook.com*
  I'm on here most days and answer members' questions.

Fitness and Nutrition Sites

- *www.FitDay.com*
  Huge site with lots of free resources available like a daily calorie tracker.

- *www.FoodFit.com*
  Great site for food calorie estimation.

- *http://health.yahoo.com/experts/eatthis*
  Eat This, Not That—entertaining and eye-opening reports on all sorts of food related topics.

- *www.bodybugg.com*
  Some patients swear by it.

Protein Supplements

- *www.Optifast.com*
  Find an Optifast provider near you.

- *www.SmartForme.net*
  Learn more about this bariatric patient-oriented food company.

Disclaimer: *This list is meant to be a guide to help readers on their weight loss journey. The information, views, and opinions presented on these websites are not necessarily endorsed by Dr. Vuong. Readers are encouraged to follow the guidelines and advice set forth by their personal healthcare providers.*

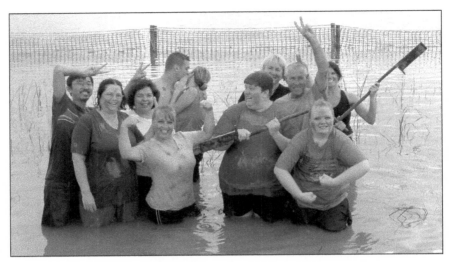

Grassplanting, October 2007—*This was our very first grassplanting with the Galveston Bay Foundation. The GBF helps preserve our wetlands by replanting cord grass and sponsoring clean ups. We were expecting to be in ankle-deep water, but the tide came in that night, so we got a lot wetter than we had planned! But it sure was fun.*

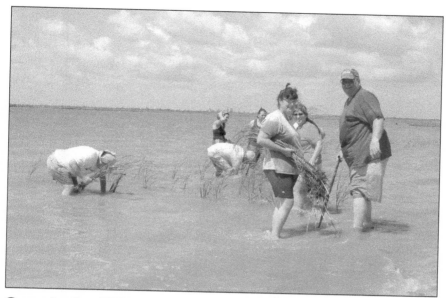

Grassplanting 5/31/08—*My patients hard at work planting grass.*

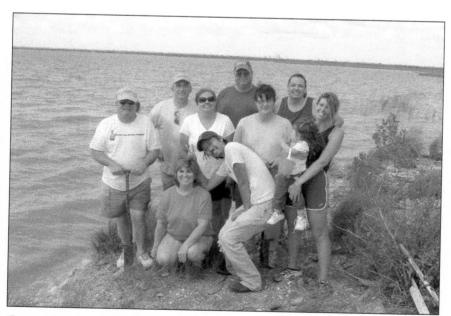

Grassplanting 5/31/08—*Another fun grassplanting. Hurricane Ike went right through this area 3 months later.*

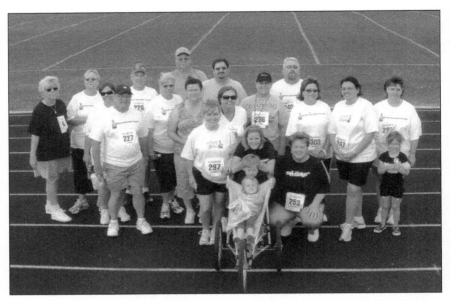

Chelseywalk, May 2008—*This is my clinic participating in the Chelsey Walk, a 5K walk to raise money for the Snowdrop Foundation. This nonprofit organization helps raise money to fight childhood cancer. Some of my patients have never walked a block much less 3.1 miles!*

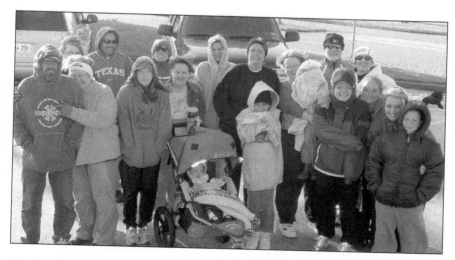

TurkeyTrot, November 2007—*This was our first TurkeyTrot. We marked out a 5K walk/jog around a local college. A cold front blew in the night before, so on Thanksgiving morning we woke to very frigid temperatures. That is why everyone is bundled up. But to my amazement, my patients still showed up! It was such a great start to our day.*

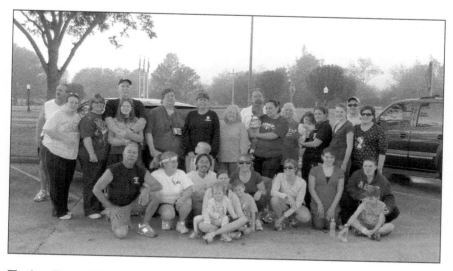

TurkeyTrot, November 2008—*We had a great turn out even though many of us didn't even have homes due to Hurricane Ike. I really believed that this event really showed the spirit of my patients.*

ABOUT THE AUTHOR

Dr. Vuong is a renowned Lap-Band surgeon from the Houston area. He received his education at Rice University, Texas A&M Medical School, completed surgical residency at St. Joseph's Hospital in Houston and currently practices in the Houston and Clear Lake areas. He is nationally recognized for his development of a successful support group program (available to patients in person and via DVD) that keeps patients on track for their long-term weight loss goals. Dr. Vuong believes that preoperative education and postoperative support groups are the key to becoming a happy, successful gastric band patient. Dr. Vuong's first book, *Tighten Your Belt: Overcome Obesity*, was well received and is considered a must read for anyone looking into gastric band surgery. He lives in the Houston area with his long time partner Melissa and their 2 and a half year old daughter, Kizzie. To learn more about Dr. Vuong please visit www.TexasCitySurgical.com and www.MoreFromMyBand.com.

Dr. Vuong also believes in giving to charity, not only as a personal philosophy, but also as a necessity for long term weight maintenance. His clinic and patients regularly participate in various fund-raiser walks and social community activities, like beach clean-ups. He has also partnered with two nonprofit organizations, the Snowdrop Foundation and the Wounded Warrior Project. The Snowdrop Foundation is a nonprofit organization that raises money to provide scholarships for college tuition to survivors of childhood cancer. The Wounded Warrior Project provides aid and empowerment for American war veterans who have been wounded in combat.

Dr. Vuong also awards free lap-band surgeries to patients who have demonstrated significant charitable giving. To find out more about this program, please visit **www.MoreFromMyBand.com.**